Yoga
the way to live

Authors
Yogachariya Jnandev Giri
Yogachariya Dr Ananda Balayogi Bhavanani

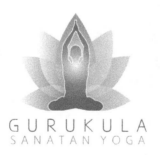

GURUKULA
SANATAN YOGA

Publisher
Design Marque

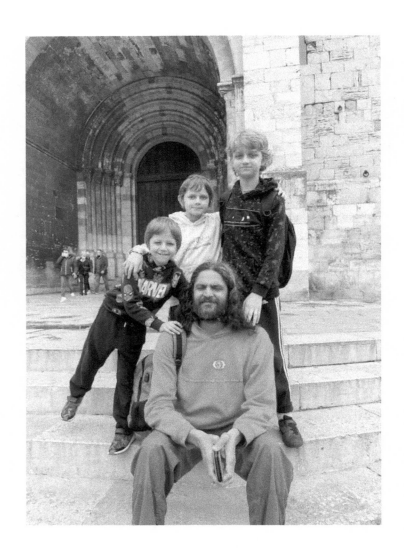

Yoga
the way to live

Authors
Yogachariya Jnandev Giri
Yogachariya Dr Ananda Balayogi Bhavanani

2022
ISBN 978-1-914485-07-7

Printed in Great Britain
by
Design Marque

Dedication

All of my ideas, thoughts and understandings about yoga and life are enriched by the teachings of Amma Meenakshi Devi, Dr Ananda and Devasana of Ananda Ashram, Puducherry, India. This book is basically based on all the aspects of yoga I have learned from various yoga and spiritual masters, literatures and institution, I am sincerely grateful to all of them for guiding me on yoga path. I am grateful to God for keeping me surrounded with loving and caring family and friends.

I am grateful to all my yoga students who keep me uplifted and motivated for teaching and reconstructing my ideas and thoughts of yogic life in western life style. I am thankful to Sarah Ray for bringing this book together with her designing skills and grateful to Mari Brame for the proof reading. I am also thankful to Yogacharini Deepika and my three children for providing me with all the support in everyday life to become who I am today.

To me yoga is my life, a way of living, and ultimate goal that I wish to succeed in life at some point. At this point in my yoga journey I feel like a beginner and I always contemplate on "if I am ever worthy of the title Yogachariya given to me by my Guru Ammaji Meenakshi Devi Bhavanani and Yogachairya Dr Ananda Balayogi Bhavanani Ji."

My heartily advice to everyone is to please try to follow each and every concept of yoga in daily life. These living teachings are not to learn or remember but they to be followed sincerely in day to day life. Success will certainly follow the one who follows the path of discipline.

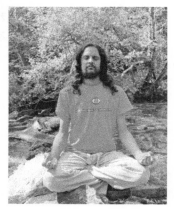

Yogachariya Jnandev Giri (Surender Saini)

Gurukula A Home of Sanatan Yoga Sadhana & Education, UK, Portugal & Online

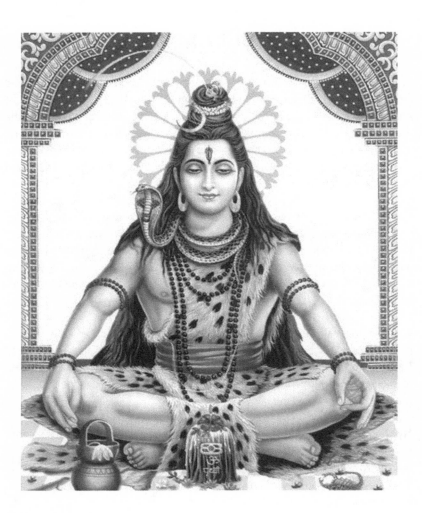

Contents

What is Yoga? 11

Yoga Scope and Classification.................................... 13

Does Living the Yoga Path Mean You Don't Have 'Fun' anymore? .. 16

The Eight Limbs of Yoga. 16

Yoga as a Life Style. 18

Finding Balance in Life-Moderate Living.................. 24

Discipline Key to Success in Life. 25

Yamas – Restraints. 28

Yamas – Beyond All Limitations. 31

Niyamas – Duties to be Adhered to for Evolution. 31

Asana – A Posture, Pose, Poise, Pause. 37

Hatha-Yoga Concept and Benefits of Asana. 39

Pranayama. 42

Pranayama is Not Only a Breathing Exercise........... 44

Basic Requirements for Good Pranayama. 47

Prana, Thoughts and Emotions.................................. 48

Prana- Philosophical Aspect....................................... 50

Naris and Pranayama.. 52

Pratyahara – Sensory Withdrawal. 55

Dharana- Concentration Practice. 57

Dhyana – Meditation.. 58

How to Meditate... 59

Samadhi- Union, Oneness, Self-Realisation............. 63

Be Aware to Avoid the Miseries Yet to Come........... 66

Yoga- Uniting the Self and Supreme Self. 67

Yoga : The Ideal Way of Life by Dr Ananda Balayogi Bhavanani.... 69

Yogachariya Jnandev 83

Yogachariya Dr. Ananda Balayogi Bhavanani 86

Yoga Moral Stories 90

Glossary 104

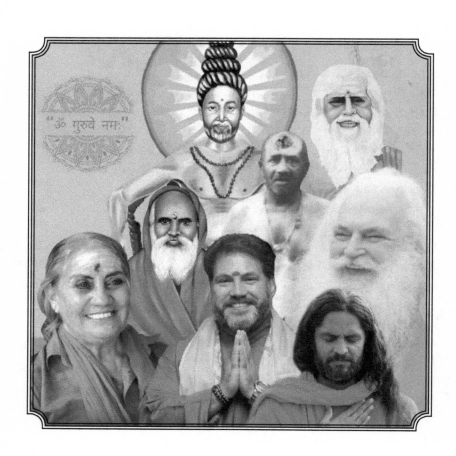

Introduction

This book is written for the Yoga sadhaka (aspirant), who is seeking to know something more of Yoga, what its roots are, where posture work fits in to the greater picture of the complete science of Yoga, as opposed to being the only purpose of Yoga. Many of the deeper philosophies and basics of yogic philosophy are addressed in this short book. It is written in a way that is easy to understand for those without any previous study of Yoga, but contains higher concepts for the more experienced yoga practitioner to contemplate.

The foundations of the yogi or yogini's spiritual life, moral and ethical considerations are addressed here, in addition to this, other forms of yoga are looked at briefly for the reader to gain some insight into the great world of yoga and how the worlds people have developed different strains of perhaps India's greatest gift, the origins of yoga. Hinduism in ancient times was very intertwined with Yogic life, as its path requires a disciplined pure lifestyle in its most refined form. When we study yoga at its roots, it is important to have some insights into ancient Hindu lifestyle which this book will include.

One of the aims of this work is to give those who already practise Yoga to develop their awareness into the higher aspects of Yoga and refine their physical practice. Yoga is essentially a tool for self development and furthermore a path to unite with the 'one' that makes up this entire universe - Yoga literally means 'union'.

I hope this book will allow you to reflect and think about your life, spiritual journey and Yoga as it has for us.

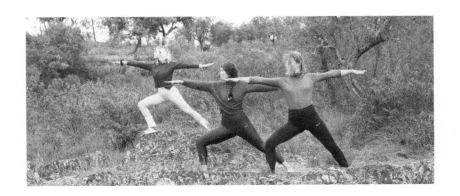

What is Yoga?

"Yoga is the science of the sciences. Yoga is an art, a philosophy, a religion, a fad and a fanaticism." The Meaning or definition of yoga depends on the individual person, according to their level of consciousness and evolution. Yoga can be simply described as the process to control the perception and the conceptions, which develop the conscious, rational thinking and viveka (discernment).

Yoga is one of most precious jewels of the Ancient Hindu ways of attaining liberation. Even then yoga is not concerned with religion. Yoga can help us to live with greater harmony. Today you can find people practising yoga everywhere. Hatha-Yoga (Asanas and Pranayama) has become the synonym of yoga. So to enhance the meaning of your life, religion, faith and practices, yoga is the tool, which is free from religion, cast or creed, available for one and all.

The term 'Yoga', which is multivalent and derived from the root 'yuj', generally means 'union', 'to join', 'to yoke together', or 'to unite as one'. The word yoga comes from the most ancient language known to man Sanskrita. In India, Sanskrit is considered to be the language of God, and is formed in a mathematical way.

Yoga in India is also considered as one of the six Ancient Indian Philosophies. Primarily we should keep in mind that yoga is the 'way of union'.

The Bhagavat-Geeta uses it (i.i.48) to mean sole desire for supreme divinity (paramesvarikaparata- sridharasvamin).

In i.i. 50 of the same treatise, yoga denotes skill in work (karmasu kausalam). In IV. 1,2,3, Yoga means Karma yoga (desire less action) and Jnanayoga (acquisition of wisdom; truth and reality).

In VI. 16, 17, the term yoga means Samadhi in which the mind is united with the Atman.

In VI. 23, yoga means a state of mind, which having realized the Supreme Being, is not disturbed even by great suffering.

In i.i. 48 and vi. 33, 36, yoga means samatva or equanimity, i.e., indifference to pleasure and pain.

Yoga can be accepted as a way of life, a way of integrating your whole awareness with the true nature of the Self. Physical, mental, emotional and spiritual aspects of your life should work in integrated harmony with each other.

In arithmetic, 'yoga' means addition. In astronomy it means conjunction, lucky conjunction and also conjunctions that may warn of danger, etc.

In the Upanishads, yoga generally means union; union of Jivatman (soul) with Parmatman (supreme soul).

Patanjali in his Yoga Sutra (i.2) defines yoga as **"yogah-chittavratti-nirodhah", this means 'to control of the whirlpools of the mind is yoga'.** By yoga, Patanjali means the effort to attain union, or oneness of Self with the Supreme Self.

What is union? In the normal sense of yoga this union means harmony of body, mind, emotions and spirit. It is living in the present, moving and accepting all situations as they are with a positive attitude.

The Devata-Smati says

"visayebhyo nivartyabhi-preterthe manasovasthapanam yogah".

Yoga means fixing the mind on the desired object.

According to Daksha-Smriti, yoga is as follows:

> **"vrittihinam manah krtva ksetrajnahparmatmani**
> **ekikrtya vimucyate yoganam mukhya ucyate."**

One who is aware of the soul, having turned the mind, which is rendered devoid of function, solely to the Supreme Soul, is liberated; this is called principal yoga.

The Vishnupurana defines yoga:
> **"atman-prayatna-sapeksa visista ya manogatih,**
> **tasya brahamani samyoga yoga ityabhidhiyate."**

The connection of that special course of mind, which depends upon ones own effort, with Brahma (The Creator) is called yoga.

Yoga- Scope and Classification

Yoga is broadly divided as Raja yoga and Hatha yoga. The former is concerned mainly with the mind and deals with various processes for controlling and calming it. Hatha yoga is concerned mainly with the body and deals with various means of keeping it fit. Several others are Mantra yoga, Laya yoga, Tantra yoga, Transcendental Meditation, Preksha Meditation, Vipsyana, etc.

1. Raja-Yoga: - Raja yoga of Patanjali, contains much of the teachings of the other systems. It aims for the self-realisation of the true nature of Purusha as absolutely distinct from Prakriti.

2. Hatha-Yoga: - It is regarded as preparatory for the practice of Raja yoga. Hatha Yoga is also a system of preventive and therapeutic asanas, kriyas, mudras and pranayamas. The term Hatha is a combination of Ha (prana) and Tha (apana). Lord Shiva in the Shiva Samhita states of 84 million asanas.

3. Mantra-Yoga: - It is the yoga of the act of repetition. This does not teach the mechanical recital of mantras. These must be preceded by earnest solitude to attain the goal and clear knowledge about the meaning of mantras. This is closely connected with the Bhakti-Yoga. The Sandilya Upanishad may be taken as a work on Mantra-Yoga. The Sivasamhita deals with the importance of mantra in practice of Yoga.

4. Laya-Yoga: - It is the yoga of absorption (laya) of mind. The Samadhi has the final aim of the realization of the identity of the finite with the supreme spirit.

5. Tantra Yoga: - Tantra yoga combines elements of both the Raja-Yoga and Hatha-Yoga with a stronger leaning towards the latter. It advocates yoga not only of meditation, but also of action. This exercise balances physical, mental and pranic/ psychic energies.

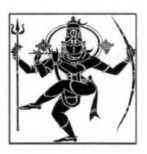

In Tantra there is no difference between Sakti (energy) and Tattva (element) so that Sakti overcomes all obstacles and brings about the unions of the yogi (yoga practitioner) with Supreme Siva. The Tantric Sadhana succeeds in weaving the microcosm and the macrocosm into a single fabric.

6. Karma Yoga: - Yoga of desireless karma (niskam - karman); Union through the action without desire. According to Swami Vivekananda, "He who goes through the streets of a big city with all the traffic and his mind is as calm as if he was in a cave, where not a sound was able to reach him; he is intensely working all the time".

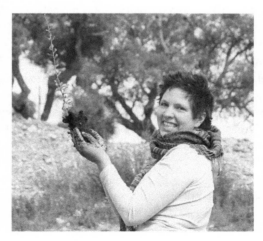

7. Jnana Yoga: - Yoga of right knowledge; union through knowledge. It has three successive stages;

1.   Viveka- discrimination between the real and non-real.
2.   Vairagya- indifference towards worldly knowledge, joy and sorrow.
3.   Mukti- liberation or union with Atman.

The yogin of the Advait Vedanta possess through successive stages in training;
·   Sravana-listening,
·   Manana- reflection on and analysis of what has been learnt
·   Nidhidhyasana- constant and profound meditation.

8. Bhakti Yoga: - In Bhakti-yoga, one devotes himself to his chosen deity to whose honour and glory every action of him is directed. According to Swami Vivekanada- "He has not to suppress any single one of his emotions; he only strives to intensify them and direct them to God". Bhakti yoga has two stages, one preparatory and other devotional.

9. Kundalini Yoga:- This includes deep study of the energy centres in the body known as the chakras. Each chakra has its own characters, shapes, color, odour, and bija (seed) sounds. The purpose of kundalini yoga is to awaken the serpent power to attain the Samadhi or moksha (freedom or liberation). This includes many kriyas, asanas, mudras, pranayamas and the chanting of bija mantras.

10. Pranayama Yoga: - Only a few pranayamas are included in traditional Hatha yoga. This school of yoga deals with controlling the prana, or the life vital force. They believe prana as the source of life. Their aim is also to activate the inactive energy sleeping in the form of the Kundalini.

However, the Gitananda Rishiculture Yoga teaches over 100 pranayamas which should be practised only after cleansing and a group of breath correcting asanas called the Hathenas.

Does living the yoga path mean you don't have 'fun' anymore?

No, of course not! To some the outer appearance of a disciplined yoga life may appear so, but once you are firmly on the yoga path it is not so in your heart, quite the opposite. Once we have refined and balanced our energies, mental and emotional layers, we need very little to feel happiness. You will not need to experience extremes to feel something!

Yoga is the control of thought-waves in the mind that are achieved by means of practice and non-attachment. Practice becomes firmly grounded when it is cultivated for a long time, uninterruptedly, with earnest devotion. Non-attachment is the exercise of discrimination that may come very slowly. But even its earliest stages are rewarded by a new sense of freedom and peace. It should never be thought of as an austerity, a kind of self-torture, something grim and painful. The practice of non-attachment gives value and significance to even the most ordinary incidents of the dullest day. It eliminates boredom from our lives. As we progress and gain increasing self-mastery, we shall see that we are renouncing nothing that we really need or want, we are only freeing ourselves from imaginary needs and desires. In this spirit, a soul grows in greatness until it can accept life's worst disasters, calm and unmoved.

The Eight limbs of Yoga (Ashtanga Yoga or Raja Yoga).

Raja Yoga or Ashtanga Yoga is known to be the highest or royal path of yoga for spiritual seekers of liberation, enlightenment or Samadhi. The eight steps or limbs of Ashtanga Yoga mentioned in the Yoga Sutras of Maharishi Patanjali are:

Yama (restraints): These are moral virtues on restraining our animal energy and desires in order to seek for peace, harmony and happiness within our individual self and community. The five Yamas are:

Ahimsa – Non-violence or non-harm

Satya – Truth or honesty

Asteya – Non-stealing or not taking anything for granted

Brahmachariya – Living in harmony with nature, discipline of sensual energy

Aparigraha – Non-greed, non-accumulation, only taking what is necessary

Niyama (observances) – These are five ethical virtues or practices to grow into a good human being and find health, peace, balance and prosperity in life. The five Niyamas are:

Saucha – Purity, cleanliness of body, space, mind, thoughts and desires

Santosha – Contentment, gratification and satisfaction with the fruits of our actions.

Tapah – Austerity, sincere practice and following the yoga path with faith and endeavour

Swadhyaya – Introspection, self-study, self-observations and acquiring knowledge from scriptures, guru and satsangas

Iswara Pranidhana – Surrendering to the divine, offering all our actions to the divine purpose, seeing divine blessing in each and every life event.

Asana (postures) – a state of being, and learning to hold our body, mind and energy still with ease. In asana we use the body as a tool to refine the subtle energies of Prana Vayus and channel them towards higher chakras.

Pranayama – refinement and enhancement of prana or vital life force, where we use the breath as a tool

Pratyahara – sensory withdrawal or withdrawal of the mind from sense objects

Dharana – concentration of mind, focusing the mind on a chosen or given single point

Dhyana – success in achieving single pointed focus, where the mind merges into a focus point; also known as meditation

Samadhi – total union of body, mind and consciousness or union of the individual self with the higher self, self-realisation, liberation, transcendental state

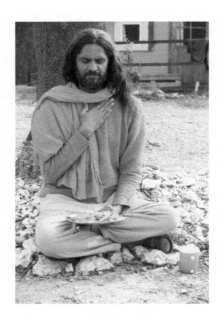

Yoga as a Life Style

Yoga is one of the most comprehensive systems, which provides us step by step tools, practices, kriyas and prakriyas, concepts and ideas, principles and code of conducts, asana and pranayama, philosophical and spiritual practices and ideas to grow physically, mentally, emotionally and spiritually.

To bring a positive change, we do need to understand our life style and the life practices that we follow. Here are a few simple questions that I would like you to ask yourself and record the answers on paper if possible.

What are the things that I do every day?

What sort of food do I eat?

What kind of drinking habits do I follow?

Do I sleep or rest enough?

Do I do enough physical exercise or not?

How do I entertain myself.

What type of social circles do I have?

What kind of work do I do?

What time do I get up and go back to bed?

These answers will give you a little idea on what kind of lifestyle you are living. Our lifestyle includes physical, mental, emotional, social, economical and spiritual activities that we take part in regularly. If you follow a sedentary life style with unhealthy food and drinking habits, you are prone to suffer with mental and physical disorders.

Foundation of yogic life style is based on Jattis, Kriyas, Asana, Pranayama and Mudra which provides balanced tools for our body, mind and soul to keep us active, healthy and balanced. Regular Hatha Yoga practice will keep you away from many physical and mental illness.

Then yoga advocates a healthy dietary habits. Eating healthy and fresh foods, vegetables, fruits, raw food, vegetarian diet, avoiding consumption of any toxic food, alcoholic drinks, drugs, smoking etc. Yogis life style describes Shaucha or purity of food, drinks, body, mind and spiritual activities and pre-conditions for health, well-being and spiritual evolution. In Ayurveda it is mentioned that "we become what we think and we are what feeds into our body".

The third important aspect of yoga is its strong foundation of ethical and moral character. Yoga teaches five Yamas (restrains) and five Niyamas (observances). As part of human life progression and evolution, we all have our basic biological needs. These are hunger, thirst and sex. These primary forces natural enforces all living beings to sustain our life and also reproduce to keep our species alive. These moral and ethical values provides us a much healthier and holistic way to fulfil our day to day needs.

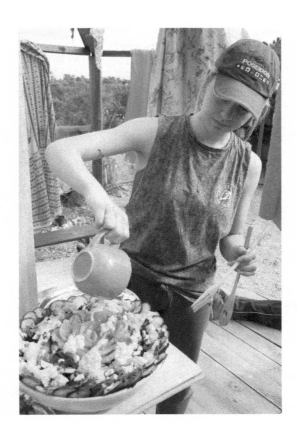

Forth Part is our Karma (actions or deeds) and Dharma (duties). We all have certain duties to fulfil. Yoga really emphasises on "attaining our true potential". We are all born with certain qualities and potentials. All the physical, mental, verbal activities that we do are classified as Karma in Yoga and Hinduism. Even our breathing, eating, sleeping, thinking, talking, etc are classified as Karma or Actions. Doing everything mindfully without worrying for fruits is one of the key Yogic idea to free ourselves from our Karmas.

Regular Practice (Tapas), Self-discipline (Anushasanam), Swadhyaya (self-awareness), Chintan and Dhyana (contemplation and meditation), Satsanga (companionships with truth seekers), Faith and devotion (Shradha and Viriya), and Iswara Prashadhana (seeing life and life events as divine blessing) are some of the key philosophical ideas that Yoga teaches us to practise in day to day life.

Key Factors to contemplate as part of healthy or Yogic life style-

Balance between exercise, rest and energy

Moral and ethical character

Healthy vegetarian diet

Cleanliness or purity of body, mind and soul

Balance, Harmony and peace within ourselves and others.

Doing our duties and taking every action mindfully.

Making every choice consciously and responsibly.

Living Mindfully for Health and Happiness

Swamiji Dr Gitananda Giriji mentions that every human being has its birth right to be healthy and happy. Further he states that everyone must claim it. Simply if you like to be healthy, you need to do everything that makes you healthy. If you like to be happy, you need to do everything that brings happiness.

As it is mentioned in Yoga and Upanishads all our unhealthy and immoral acts have their roots in Avidya or ignorance. Ignorance is not only not knowing the truth or what is right to do, but it is also not following the truth or practices we know that are good for our health and happiness.

We all have a natural force in, which has the pleasure seeking principle. This enforces us to do many things that our Viveka (reasoning) and Buddhi (intellect) tells us not to do in certain way or situations or guides us a much more healthier way to fulfil our desires. We all have the intuition which is sometimes known as gut-instinct. To empower this, we must live mindfully.

In day to day life, we all wake up, do daily tasks, eat, drink, go to work, talk to family and friends, social media, and many other activities without even knowing, as daily habits. Yogic or mindful living advocates in an awareness of the activities that we take part in every day. Every choice we make from waking up to eating, drinking, working, sleeping, entertainment, etc should be a conscious choice.

If we can be mindful of every activity that we follow, it will naturally bring balance and appreciation. We tend to always act or respond better when we are aware of the situation. Our prana or energy flows where our mind goes. Hence if we start doing things consciously, our energy will flow into the right parts of body and mind. Let's say, if you are eating and also watching television, your body has to decide where to supply the most energy. Naturally if you are eating, excess energy should be supplied to your mouth, slavery glands, and stomach. But if you are also watching something, then the priority becomes our brain. This will lead to many digestive problems.

This mindful living also allows us to appreciate day to day activities, which normally many people don't value much like eating, resting, social times, entertainment, etc. Many people have such big ambitions that they don't have a moment to care for their body, mind and soul.

Simple Mindful Activities-

Sit down enjoy every sip of your cup of tea or coffee.

Go for a walk and enjoy every step and details.

Make time to relax or meditate and let go of everything else for few minutes.

While you eating your meals, focus on your food and enjoy the flavours.

Light a candle or incense that you like and enjoy the fragrance.

Play your favourite music and try to be fully absorbed in it.

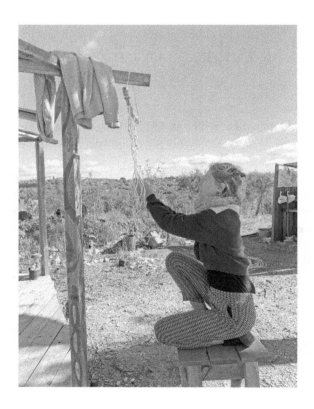

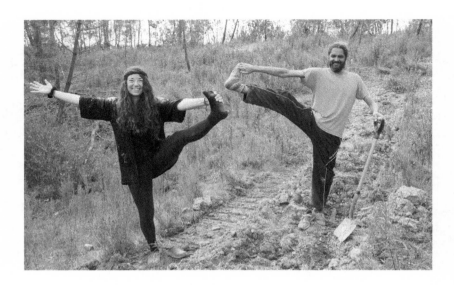

Finding Balance in Life- Moderate Living

Balance is very important in life. As Lord Krishna mentions in Bhagavat Gita "Yoga is Equanimity (yoga samatva ujyate)." But how do we attain this balance or harmony. Lord Krishna further states that to be successful in Yoga or any other aspect of life, we need to follow things moderately. He mentions that "one who eats too much, or not eating enough, one who exercise too much or not doing enough exercise, one who works too much or not working enough, one who sleeps too much or not sleeping enough will never succeed in life."

This clearly gives us healthy guidelines on working on our own health, well-being and spiritual evolution. If you're not eating enough, you will have no energy to fulfil all your Dharma or duties and take part in day to day tasks. On the other hand if we eat too much that causes toxicity and burden on our digestive system, and liver. This may result into obesity, lethargy and heaviness of body and mind.

If are not doing enough physical activities, work and exercise, we are prone to suffer with stiffness, physical weakness, joint immobility, arthritis, blood and heart problems. Not doing our duties may also result in family, social and economic problems. Overdoing things, exercise or work will cause exhaustion and tiredness, which will also result in many physical, mental and emotional health issues.

Sleep is another important aspect of our life. A healthy sleep allows our body to heal, rejuvenate and prepare for another day of activities and tasks. Sedantary life style, sleeping too much may result in physical problems like obesity, muscle and joints pain, heart problems, depression, anxiety, stress and lack of self-confidence.

The Key idea is very simple and profound here- "live your life in harmony or balance between your energy, action and rest." So if your work demands physical activities, then you need to eat more than some one who has a less physical demanding job. If your job demands mental activities, then you must find time to do physical exercise, relaxation and meditation.

Discipline Key to Success in Life

Patanjali begins explaining yogic journey of self-realisation with the first yoga sutra stating "Yoga as a Path of Discipline" (atha yoga anushasanam). It also tell us that we all have the potential to attain success in field of yoga or any other goal in life, if we are willing to go inward and find the answers as well as do what needs to be done. There is always a deeper meaning and reason to everything that is around us or happening in our life. We just need to look deep within and follow the path with the right attitude.

For many of us these days discipline seems to be a negative term. The moment we say that I have to follow something, our mind starts to debate against it. We are all looking for freedom. We like to be living under a free will. We like to do, what we like to do or feel like doing. But we keep forgetting that we can only be free by following discipline in our life. If we do everything as it should be done, with the right intention, attitude and intellect, we are free. We are all individuals and need to look after our individual health, well-being and happiness. But we are also collective beings, and hence we have to be mindful of everyone around us.

Patanjali beings with the word 'ATHA' which literally means "here and now". Living here and now and paying attention to the right now and not in the past or future. It can also be seen as it is for 'I' or 'You' or the one who follows. So if you follow this discipline, here and now, you will be benefited.

The word ANU from anushasanam means "atom" — the smallest or minute, the which cannot be broken further and that which makes the WHOLE. This whole universe is composed from various forms of atoms. Word Shasanam means ruling or governing. Atom can be seen as the subtlest form of our existence and energy while Shasanam is to govern or master this true essence or Nature. Anushasnam is Sanskrita means Discipline of our body, and mind actions. Anushashnam or discipline is live in harmony with our true NATURE AND ESSENCE. It is our Dharma or duty to look after our health and well-being and grow in our life, hence 'anushasanam is to do everything that we need to do in order to attain health, well-being, happiness and spiritual evolution.

When we live in the here and now and follow all the discipline with great humane virtues of honesty, love, compassion, forgiveness, self-awareness and live in deeply harmony with our true nature, it opens the doors to limitless possibilities.

There are natural laws of geometry bringing harmony, dynamic life transformations and beauty which we can see through flowers, butterflies, birds, plants, fruits, animals, trees, planets, starts, moon, sun, etc. We can see how alive the whole universe is and how much harmony and dynamic dance of energy exists. Living here and now with discipline will bring us this whole dynamic harmony, and peace in us. Our life will become full of joy, abundance and love.

The discipline here and now is to also appreciate everything that we have in our life. It is to respect, value and be grateful. Whenever we are living in past or future we suffer mentally and emotionally for what we don't have or couldn't get, or fearful of getting in future. We are so obsessed about exploiting our resources, nature, mother earth to make our life comfortable or gain power and wealth. Yogic attitude and virtues will enable us to look deep within the laws of nature and live in harmony within our own true nature and with external universal living and non-living beings.

Remember, if you are planning to go for an adventure, or journey, where will you start. You have to start your journey from where you are. Once you begin your journey, to get to your destination, you need to follow the right path and you need to also follow it till you get there. If you want to reach the top of a mountain, you must keep climbing up as well as choose the right path and prepare yourself for the journey.

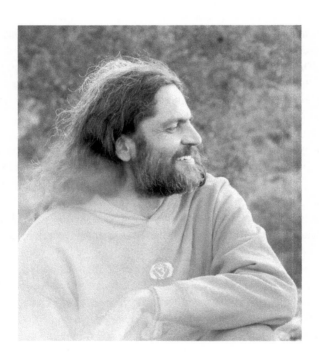

Yamas ~ Restraints

A strong building can only be built up on a strong foundation. If your foundation is weak, your building will collapse very soon. The same rule is applicable to the yogic approach of spiritual evolution. If your base of moral character, behaviour, attitude, thoughts, beliefs, emotions and finally physical actions are not right or correct, you can not grow on the path of yogic evolution. These days most of the modern yogic teachings avoid the importance of Yamas and Niyamas. In ancient times in India, you must have perfected these to some degree before you were allowed to study under a Yoga Master.

Swamiji Dr. Gitananda Giri Gurumaharajaji says that yamas and niyamas are the basic foundations of yogic evolution. Without perfecting them one cannot attain the highest stage of purity, bliss and joy. Yamas and niyamas are not optional in yoga; their perfection is not only needed but is essential for all yoga sadhakas (truth seekers).

In a yogic perspective, yama/niyama are not ends or goals in themselves, nor are they rules nor prescriptions, but merely remedial processes designed to help us to grow on the path of evolution of the inner eternal law (Sanatana Dharma).

Yamas are restraining our animal nature and then through the Niyamas we change lower energy to the higher energy of love, compassion, and respect for all.

In Hinduism 'Yama' is also known as the lord of death and death is unavoidable for all the living beings. Thus yamas should be followed and perfected like the ultimate goal in life and one can attain the highest stage of yogic evolution only through perfection of the yamas and niyamas. One may break down the word, yama, in an unconventional way; 'ya' meaning that which moves, while 'ma' represents the mother principle: nature's/creation's nurturing principle. Thus in this analysis yama means to bring forth, nurture and move with the natural processes of creation. Death is an unavoidable truth of your birth.

The five Yamas are:
Ahimsa-satya-asteya-brahmacarya-aparigraha yamah. (Yoga-sutra. II 30.)

1.   **Ahimsa** non-violence, i.e. the removal of violence from our own life as well as others taken in the non-dual sense, or that we are all one. This also includes protecting our own body and personal space from harm.

2.   **Satya** truthfulness being the removal of the veils of deceit and falsehood from our lives including that of self deception.

3.   **Asteya** honesty, non-stealing, non-exploitation of others, and integrity in all our relations.

4.   **Brahmacharya** continuity, centeredness, wedded-ness, or one-pointedness to the all inclusive weave of "Source" - harmony and union in true Integrity while not allowing oneself to be distracted from the spiritual goal. Control of our energy.

5.   **Aparigraha** non-possessiveness, non-greed, non-envy, non-attachment, letting go, non-false identification penetrating throughout the mind in meditation as well as in all our relationships as the simplification of our life so that we are better able to focus on the spiritual goal latent in every moment.

Each Yama and Niyama could fill a book individually, but for a little insight I have expanded more. Yamas and Niyamas all have their root in ahimsa (not harming living beings); their aim is to perfect this love that we ought to have for all creatures.

Ahimsa, or non-violence is not harming or supporting any harmful activity to any one or the self through our thoughts, emotions and actions. Since everybody on the planet has caused some harm to other animal forms or plants, the spiritual truth that ahimsa points to is simply to more deeply commune and inter-connect with the practices of non-violence, not harming others or self, and actually removing harm to others (healing) and self especially in the transpersonal sense where "the other" and the self are one in our daily actions so that balance and continuity in our authentic yoga practice is accelerated and realised.

Satya or truth is being adhered to the truth and reality in all situations. Satya is also behaving righteously to save and protect the dharmas and humanity. In the yogic aspect satya is also to teach and speak about the yogic approaches and spirituality you have experienced and not by listening or reading from books.

It is not so concerned with "telling the truth" externally as much as it is in its inner (antar) esoteric meaning of removing the ingrained Samskaras which support self deceit and conceit.

In simple definition Samskaras are deep imprinted positive values of life in your personality. While in yogic perspective these are bondages of your positive and negative karmas/deeds in present and previous lives. To grow up on this spiritual path you have to work out all of them and there is no shortcut in the yoga path.

Thus satya should be practised with the body, speech, and mind. Satya thus does not mean to restrain deceit as much as to bring forth Truth; i.e., to remove falsehood, confusion, illusion, delusion, and ignorance.

Brahmachariya as merely the sexual restraint is a misunderstanding of its practice and great values. Brahmachariya in its vast meanings is to adhere with the natural laws or the universal laws of this creation of Brahma. Brahmacharya is to reveal, acknowledge, and act in accordance with the eternal inner eternal teacher. Brahmacharya is practiced thus not as a restraint of the body, but within the integration of the body, speech, and mind as an affirmation of a way of life.

Asteya is not only non-stealing of material things, but also includes time, peace, privacy, and even thoughts. It is being honest in all aspects of individual as well as social life. Positive attitude, gratitude and being grateful to your parents, friends, and teachers for helping you or providing all these resources and knowledge are part of practising Asteya. On an universal level caring for nature and not exploiting mother earth's resources is Asteya.

Aparigraha is not only to eliminate exploitation, contradiction, deceit, self dishonesty, greed, attachment, and selfishness, but to act to promote integrity, honesty, generosity, trust, abundance, fulfilment, and gratefulness, contentment, and clarity in body, mind and speech. Aparigraha is living your life with the minimum resources you need to live a healthy and happy life rather than accumulating everything even if you don't need them and can be used by others. This can help us to save the planet from environmental catastrophe.

Yamas ~ Beyond All Limitations

Jati-desa-kala-samaya-anavacchinnah sarva-bhauma maha-vratam (yoga-sutra. II 31.)

The above sutra means : adhering to these Yamas in all situations, at all times, without limitations or exceptions will turn the tide effecting closure of and sealing off the great gate of death and dissolution, thus moving us into greater synchronization with the natural laws of the universe as it is (Sanatana Dharma).

This sutra emphasizes the practice of all the yamas in each and every situation and not only with certain people or in certain situations. Yamas should be perfected with all the living races, in all the places and states, and at all times. One can attain the highest stage only by perfecting the yamas, only then can we attain freedo'm from the cycle of life and death. Practicing yamas with body, mind and emotions with each and every situation is the way of cleansing out your past karmas and bondages of the karmas.

It is seen that the root of all the sins is the bhaya, or fear and clinging to life of the survival instincts at any cost (abhivinasha). Thus one should try to develop detachment, as in Lord Krishna's teaching in the Geeta that "you do your duty without desiring for the fruits." Swami Vivekananda also emphasized that to develop all the humane values you need to be fearless. So be fearless! Be fearless!

Thus yamas are to protect the inner as well as outer self, or real self which is a part of Mother Nature. These should be perfected in reference of human beings, animals, plants and the environment. If you are damaging the real or true form of nature, this is violence or untruthful behaviour for our upcoming generations.

Niyamas~ Duties to be Adhered to for Evolution

'Ni', means that which is inherent or underneath. As such the niyamas clarify, complement, and expand upon the yamas. The niyamas thus are even more proactive actions that Patanjali encourages us to undertake in order to accelerate one's success in yoga. Yama and niyama are both leading to the same destination. For example, ahimsa and satya promote saucha and swadhyaya, asteya and aparigraha lead to santosha and tapas, brahmacharya leads to isvara pranidhana, while the reverse is also true; i.e., that the practice of the niyama leads to the realization of the yamas.

After restraining the animal instincts by perfecting the yamas you come to the point of building up human nature and this starts with the practice of the niyamas in yoga. All animal instincts are inborn characteristics in all of us. The human nature has to be encouraged in us. This work starts with the teachings in family by our parents, grandparents, relatives, society and school. They teach us naturally how to behave with our body, mind and emotions and then how to behave properly with others in different situations. So if you will do swadhyaya you will find that the foundation of all the yamas is being made from the first day of your life when you started to learn.

1. Saucha on a gross physical level is the obvious general cleanliness of the body and appearance as well as abstaining from poisoning the body or burdening it with food and drinks that it can not be digested, assimilated, or eliminated easily. This will unburden not only the digestive system, but the elimination and immune systems thus creating more available energy for the process of evolutionary higher consciousness to unfold. Another inner application of Saucha is keeping the manomaya kosha (mental thoughts / energy body) free from all the negativities. So in normal life keeping your body, mind, emotions on an individual level and then cloths, surroundings, and environment on an external level is Saucha.

Saucha may be applied to our belief systems whether or not they may be tainted, and thus be a source of taint, impurity, and affliction to our consciousness (until purified). In this sense transformation and rebirth is an action of purification. Yet another manifestation of Saucha is in our motivations and actions. But since actions follow thought and consciousness (or lack thereof) it seems that the purification of consciousness is more significant to this process.

2. Santosha is contentment, fulfilment, completion, and peace. As such it denotes abundance (not scarcity), happiness (not discontent), and in a deeper sense especially deep gratitude. By gratitude, one does not need to be grateful to any person or event, but rather it is the deep heartily felt sense of unconditional gratitude.

Santosha is practised as peace and happiness as love. We commune with peace and abundance and give it forth- manifest it. When greed, lust, conflict, war, trickery, competition, himsa (violence), pain, theft, deceit, corruption, falsity, and ignorance are defeated; when the invincible Supreme Self is victorious; then Santosha reigns supreme! In the meanwhile we must attempt to assess our allegiance with grief, war, conflict, anger, hatred, jealousy, hurt, and fear; be willing to surrender them and to alter them to peace and lasting happiness.

'Kriya yoga'... Niyamas continued

Patanjali states that one can directly attain the samadhi or oneness only through perfecting the three niyamas- tapas, swadhyaya and isvar-pranidhan. These three together are also termed as kriya-yoga (this does not refer to the Kriya Yoga of Paramhansa Yoganananda).

3. Tapas is not simply renunciation, but rather a recycling of the energy that could have been placed into further distraction and dissipation; placing this energy into one's spiritual evolution. Tapas becomes the activity that freshens up and sparks a practice that has become sluggish and dull. As such then it is an affirmation of the higher Self. This is the action of authentic tapas. Very simply by letting go of one's attachment in such neurotic activities or propensities, then space and energy is liberated and reclaimed that can now be directed toward pure essence or supreme self.

4. Swadhyaya is not merely "scriptural study" or book study. Although studying "right spiritual" philosophy and practising contemplation on mental and psychological phenomena (jnana yoga) can provide some specific benefits of clarification or insight to higher aspects. Such external study can be often very misleading and disorientating (unless balanced with inner study).

Thus in a yogic sense swadhyaya means studying, observing, and eventually knowing our true self nature, not through the conceptual confines and objective externalized eyes of the intellect, books, scripture, or authority, but rather through Gnosis acquired through meditation; from an authentic direct transpersonal experience. This study or inquiry into Self is an essential practice of the process of self realisation via the removal of delusion/illusion (maya).

5. Isvara is often mistranslated with the English term, "God", which in the Western sense of the term, is almost the opposite of what is meant because Isvara specifically is not a theistic idea (as yoga is not theistic). In other words the word Isvara specifically refers to the formless and deity-less, "aspectless aspect" of the divine aspect of Reality in Yoga. Thus Isvara pranidhana is to surrender to the great integrity of formless infinity which is the eternal (beginning-less and ending-less). The word, Isvara, thus expresses or symbolizes completeness, the whole or infinite mind and as such cannot be represented by symbols being the nothingness that includes everything.
The following four verses of yoga sutras clarify all the misleading thoughts regarding the Isvara-

Klesha-karma-vipakasayair apara-mrshta purusa-visesa isvarah (Sutra 24)- Isvara is the purest (a-para-mrshta) aspect (visesa) of pure undifferentiated universal consciousness (purusa) which is untouched and unaffected by taint (klesha), karma, and the seed germs (asayair) that result (vipaka) from ordinary desire and propensities.

Tatra-nir-atishayam sarvajna-bijam(Sutra 25) -There (tatra) [isvara] is the seed and origin (bija) of absolute (nir-atishayam), unsurpassed, and complete omniscience (sarvajna).

Tasya vachakah pranavah(Sutra 27) - Isvara is expressed and represented (vachakah) by the vibratory energy contained in the pranava (the sacred syllable, om).

Taj-japas tad-artha-bhavanam(Sutra 28) - Through generating (bhavanam) constant repetition (taj-japa) of the pranava (om) the meaning (artha) behind the sound is realised and becomes manifest (bhavanam).

In the "Geeta" Lord Krishna says: "Many are the means described for the attainment of the highest goal....but love is the highest of all; love and devotion that make one forget everything else; love that merge the devote with me...as all earthly pleasure fade into nothingness." The path of love is considered supreme because it is wholly selfless and eternal the total erasing of self for the love of the Supreme Self. The chains of desire bind us. The Jnani's strength and knowledge breaks the chains; the Bhakta, on the other hand, becomes so small and ego-less they slip through the chains. In bhakti, the mind melts in love for God and so is dissolved in Supreme Soul. In Jnana, the mind is mastered and over-powered by the force of wisdom. The same is described in the following three verses of the yoga sutras:

Samadhi-siddhir Isvara-pranidhanat(II 45.)-Samadhi is perfected (siddhir) through letting go the limited matrix of a separate self while surrendering to isvara (the all inclusive aspectless and unconditioned great universal integrity or the underlying motive power behind the principle of Infinite Mind).

Sauca-samtosa-tapah-svadhyaya-isvara-pranidhanani   niyamah (II 32.) - Niyama consists of saucha (purity), santosha (contentment and peacefulness), tapas (spiritual passion and fire), swadhyaya (self study and mastery), and Isvara pranidhana (surrender to the Universal Great Integrity of Being).

Tapah-svadhyayesvara-pranidhanani   kriya-yogah(II.1) -   Tapas (spiritual passion, energy, or heat generated through forgoing dissipative activities), swadhyaya (self study), and isvara pranidhana (the function of surrender to or the embrace of the all encompassing comprehensive integrity which interconnects us all (who we really are) are the three essential prerequisite (kriya) activities that lead us to realizing the fruit of yoga.

Sri Sathya Sai Baba says; "love is the most powerful thing in the world.... All the yogas are included in the path of the love, and whoever attains this love, attains God."

Mystics and Saints of all religions have testified the beauty of supreme love. 'It is the power that makes the sun and stars to move' said Dante. According to scriptures, God created this universe for love and that love is the very purpose of our existence. Love confirms Ananda/Bliss and softens the grind of mundane existence.

Tyagraj sang: "Is there greater Bliss O God, than to dance, to sing to you, to pray for your presence, and unite with you in my mind?" The Narada Bhakti

Sutras describe Bhakti as a transcendental experience of bliss, in which the ego is completely dissolved and absorbed, in the Supreme Soul.

Love is without boundaries and ever expanding, like God, who is limitless. The love of Gopis (lovers) for Krishna is celebrated in our scriptures because of its glorious nature. Such love transcends mind and the body and touches the soul.

Divine love is free from any motive. Divine love is transitory, a pure reflection of the real thing. Worldly love is erratic and subject to change; but love for God is unchanging and eternal, everlasting. Divine love is perfect, it is always charged with its own energy. It is nitya- nautnam or fruitful and ever new.
To attain this state, however, we have to pay a price. Meera Bai, 16th century Saint-Poet, sang: "Kanha, the price He asked, I gave. Some cry, I gave in full, weighed to the utmost grain, my love, my life, my soul, my all...." As mystics have testified there is peace and fulfilment in devotion that nothing else can bring.

A devotional prayer with total devotion for the supreme self.

"I pray not for wealth,
I pray not for ownership,
I pray not for pleasures or even for the joys of poetry.
I only pray that during all my life,
I may have love:
That I may have love to God

The incorporation of these yamas / niyamas into our daily lives will serve as guideposts to show us where we go astray and where we can better connect more completely and continuously with the Source. These guidelines of ahimsa, truthfulness, integrity, non-possessiveness, continuity, purity, peacefulness, divine passion, self study, and surrender can also be expediently applied to our daily asana practice to accelerate to its highest accomplishment as well.

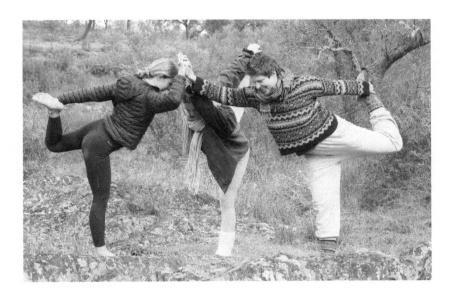

Asana – A Posture, Pose, Poise, Pause

Asana is another beautiful Sanskrita term which has many meanings. On our yoga mat, asana means a posture, pose or practice to control our body, mind and subtle energies in order to master our inner self. Asana is a key part of Hatha Yoga and modern yoga. Sadhaka or practitioners can perform asana in a very gentle and static manner, for restoration. They can also practise extreme dynamic vinyasa or flow for strength, flexibility, endurance, health and vitality.

Patanjali mentions Asana as the third limb of Ashtanga Yoga after Yamas and Niyamas. He simply defines Asana as "a state of being at ease with stability within our individual self." He further mentions that Asana can also be practised with effort and ease, and that the sadhaka should try to relax while performing Asana. This leads a hatha yoga sadhaka to a state of equanimity and discipline of body, mind, energy and senses.

Krishna in the Bhagavad Gita explains that "a yoga sadhaka must sit in a comfortable posture, with erect spine, and hold that posture with ease whilst focusing the mind at the tip of the nose and watch the breath, in order to master the mind."

A comfortable asana or seat is the pre-requisite for inner or advanced yoga practices (antaranga yoga). The Upanishads and Hatha Yoga scriptures mention that a sadhaka should practise asana in a clean, secluded and tranquil place on a clean floor or piece of ground covered with straw, wool, or a cotton rug. It is also mentioned that "one should learn asana from a Guru who has obtained realisation" and "should never use them for demonstration or showing off on purpose."

Hatha Yoga and Trantra Yoga mentions 84 million postures and further states that out of those 84 are more important asanas or yonis. Out of all those, four meditation postures (dhyansana) are known to be most important, being mentioned in various Yoga scriptures. These are:

Sukhasana – an easy cross-legged position

Vajrasana or Bhadrasana – the thunderbolt position, sitting on heels

Siddhasana – the perfect pose

Padmasana – the lotus pose

Swastikasana – the auspicious pose

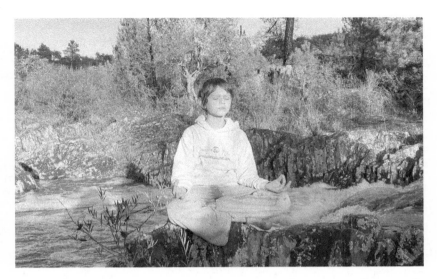

Hatha-Yoga Concept and Benefits of Asanas

Hatha yoga and all the Tantric practices are based on the concept of the loma-viloma. The Sanskrita word 'hatha' is derived from the joining of 'ha' and 'tha'. 'Ha' is the solar energy represented by the warm golden sun. 'Tha' is the lunar energy represented by the cool silvery moon. The aim of all the hatha yoga and tantric practices is union and balancing of the 'ha' and 'tha'; solar and lunar energies, within the body.

The right part of the body is represented by the masculine characters of shiva and the left half body is representation of the feminine characters of shakti. This sun and moon; warm golden and cool silvery; ha and tha; energies are known as loma and viloma respectively. These are also represented by the prana and apana energies.

Prana moves from the top to the bottom in the right half of the body while stapana moves from the bottom to the top in the left half of the body. This is also found in the concept of the polarity of the human body. Energy always flows in the wide oval shape in and out side the body.

Our human life is a representation of five bodies, or panch-koshas. These are annamaya kosha, or the physical body; pranamaya kosha or the psychic body; manomaya kosha or the mental body; anadamaya kosha or the blissful body; vijnanamaya kosha or the pure subtle body or the soul. The loma and viloma energies are manifestation of the positive energy and the negative energy from the subtle to the gross body.

The process of human evolution from the animal nature to the human nature and then to the purest nature of super conscious is from the gross or the physical body. Body awareness and awareness of the loma and viloma energies refines and purifies these energies to their subtle forms to gain the harmony and oneness with the self and nature.

The five gross pranas, apana, vyana, prana, samana and udana flow in various parts of our body in various directions to keep the physical, mental and emotional process in health and harmonious functioning. They regulate the normal functioning of the body area they are concerned with.

Asanas are designed to align the body skeletal system. These strengthen the legs, thighs, pelvic area muscles, and shoulders.

Asanas reduce the fat of the hips, thighs, and abdomen and west region. These are also good for directing the blood flow to the inner parts of the knees, thighs, and lower back region and thus eradicate the toxins accumulated there.

It directs the blood flow towards the heart and lungs and thus prevents the chances of developing any coronary and heart diseases. All sections of the lungs are activated and reproduced. They also provide a very good message to the digestive organs and increase the digestive fire.

Postures are also of high importance in the spiritual aspects as most of the shapes of the asanas are related to our psychic energy centres, charkas, e.g. triangle shape / Trikanasana.

Asanas also reverse the blood flow and pranic energy in the body. They also generate the sensitivity and awareness of the whole body muscles and organs and thus are of great importance to practise concentration and especially shavasana (yogic relaxation pose) and the yoga-nidra. Shavasana and yoga-nidra are pre-requisite for meditation.

Asanas are aimed to align the body skeletal system. Whole body joints are loosened and this increases their mobility. Bones are strengthened and their rigidity is removed. This prevents the bone decomposition and thus keeps us fit until old age. Asanas contain various forward and back stretching positions which help to balance our energies;
The silvery cool apana moves from bottom to the top of the body. This is also known as shakti or the feminine energy in all human beings. Prana moves from the top of the body to the bottom. This golden prana is also known as shiva, or masculine energy.

According to Maharishi Patanjali, "sthiram sukham asanam" which means a firm, and comfortable position is asana or posture. Here Maharshi states that a firm and pleasing position in which sadhaka can sit for higher spiritual practices is known as asana.

In the Bhagavad-Gita Lord Krishna states that a sadhaka in asana should sit with an erect spine neck and head then gaze constantly at the tip of the nose and contemplate ME (God).

According to Shiva-samahita there are 84 million postures and asanas which are associated with the yoni or creation or different species. Many asanas presently are associated with birds and animals such as matsyasana (fish posture), mayurasana (peacock posture), bakasana (herring), mandukasana (frog), etc.

In authentic scriptures of Hatha-yoga 32 asanas are mentioned. Four of them are most important – Sukkha asana (pleasant pose), Padma asana (lotus pose), Varjra asana (thunderbolt pose), Siddha asana (perfect pose).

Presently the meaning of asanas is changed and expanded. Now asanas are used for strength, stamina and health promotion. Normally yoga is considered as merely a few asanas and pranayamas. Asanas are often performed in acrobatic style to maintain a slim and beautiful body.

In ancient times asanas were practised for transforming the lower sexual energy into a higher spiritual energy. It was aimed to balance the pancha-koshas, pancha-pranas and shiva-shakti or loma-viloma energy aspects.

The aim of all yogic practices is unity of both the feminine and masculine energies in our body to attain the oneness or union of the self with the supreme self. Asanas have a complete approach to transverse the apana and prana in the middle anahata chakra for the union or merging into each other. It refines the gross prana to the subtle pure prana, which is essential to realize the higher aspects of yogic practices.

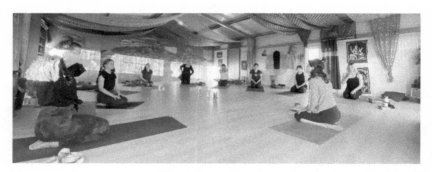

Pranayama

Pranayama yoga is the "science of breath", the control of the vital force (prana) present in the air we breath. The Sanskrita term pranayama means: 'Prana' is the divine universal creative energy or power, and the 'yama' means control or the science of control.

The word 'prana' can be broken further as 'pra' meaning to exist independently, or to have the prior existence. 'Ana' is the shortened term for 'anna' meaning a cell, or collectively 'ana'. Thus 'prana' means "that which existed before any atomic or the cellular life came into being". Such life is termed as manifestation of the divine.

Behind all the manifestation of creation and life is this divine energy prana. Most of the prana we receive is from the air we inhale. But we also receive it to some extent from water and food. Some part is also absorbed directly in the skin from the atmosphere.

Remember that the prana is not oxygen or the other gases we inhale nor the nutrients we take from the food. The truth is that behind using all these nutrients and the gases for breathing this divine energy prana plays the role as the catalyst. Prana is absorbed through the exposed nerve endings of the body and especially in the nostrils, mouth and back of the throat. Thus eat slowly and chew properly to allow the releasing and absorbing of the prana. Water should be sipped slowly to allow the absorption of prana in the throat and mouth.

We must learn pranayama from the beginning to do Dirgha Pranayama, deep slow and controlled breath. Most of us nowadays are shallow breathers and lacking the prana or the oxygen for the normal functioning of our body, mind and emotions. Most of the present diseases are the result of improper breathing. All illnesses can be alleviated by practising pranayama properly and by attaining perfection in them. For a yogi the breathing should be under the total awareness. This conscious breathing brings the autonomic functions under the control of the nervous system or the will.

Improper breathing, dyspnoea or laboured breathing is not a recent problem. But now it becomes more prominent because of a stressful lifestyles and the adverse environmental conditions making it worse. Even Yogi Gorakshanatha travelled the whole of the India and gave the message-

"O men and women of India! You have defaulted from the good health by being the shallow breathers".

He stated that in his age people were breathing only one-eighth of their capacity. He cured many of the diseases only by teaching the asanas and pranayamas.

When we do shallow breathing, the nerve receptors sited deep in the lungs are unaffected. Only when we breathe in and out deeply these inspiratory and expiratory receptors get stimulated and called for their desired activity. This sends the reflexo-genic feed-back to the brain. This governs the control over the in and out breath along with the hold in and the hold out breath.

Breath is also related to our life and spirit or the soul. Even it is said that there is life in the body, if there is breath in the body. In Sanskrita word Brahman is used for the breath. In taking the breath is termed as inspiration in Greek, which comes from 'in-spiro' means being in tune with the spirit or the God. While expiration is originated from the 'ex-piro' means to be out of the spirit. In India if some one dies they say in Hindi 'prana tyaga diye' which means literally that 'prana left the body'.

The yogis performed the pranayamas and found that they can fulfil their need of prana only through the air with no other sustenance. They don't need to eat food and are known as breatharians. Still there are yogis in various parts of the world who are alive without food and even some are without water.

Pranayama is Not only a Breathing Exercise

Simply a yogic practice called pranayama where one starts by first taking firm and pleasant asana (sthirama-sukham-asanam), then turning attention upon the inhalation and exhalation of the breath in order to extend and refine (ayama) the prana. According to Patanjali **Pranayama is an awareness/ observation practice, not a mechanical practice.**

First you all should know that the most common mistranslation- "pranayama is the control or regulation of the inhalation, exhalation, and retention of breath". Then in this case we should call it 'swashayama'.

The first misinterpretation of the word, prana, as breath, which makes the definition redundant as well as misleading. Pranayama is the extension, spreading, thinning, refinement, or expansion of energy, where prana is life energy and "ayama" is expansion, thinning, rarefaction, or extension.

The definition of yama as control or regulation, reflects concepts of hatha yoga which believed that liberation could be attained through forcefulness and control of the body, breath, and mind. Similar mistranslations: nirodha as control, tapas as self abnegation, swadhyaya as scriptural study, or brahmacharya as sexual restraint where there exists no objective or experiential basis.

We have to learn to expand and refine the prana by observing and breaking apart the movements of the breath as it occurs in inspiration and expiration so that it is no longer controlled by the unconscious winds of karma, thoughts, emotions and unconscious habits, but rather it comes into the light of awareness. In this way our energy and mind changes as well as our karma.

Pranayama can be started first as the process (gati) of becoming aware of our vital energy by breaking it down into its gross external components as manifest in the profound linkages between mind and energy inherent in the breathing process. Try to inculcate the awareness of how the energy enters our body/mind, how it leaves it, and how it becomes discontinuous or inhibited. Then we obtain awareness of how the energy is extended, refined, and made more subtle so that we open up the nadis (the flows of the prana) which activates the body's higher potential.

Prana (with a capital "P" permeates all of the Universe without it nothing moves, but also prana with a small "p" denotes the vital energy (prana) as it permeates the physical body. It is strongly associated with the breath as the animating principle- as the sustained-linking creation with Infinite Source. Indeed breathing is the most primal activity of human life. Breath performs a bridge between the unconscious (autonomic) and conscious (central) nervous systems. In hatha. kundalini, and tantra yoga pranayama is not just a powerful awareness tool, but a focused practice capable of balancing and synchronizing not only the autonomic and central nervous systems, but also the afferent and efferent nervous systems and the sympathetic and parasympathetic nervous systems as all polarities can be accessed through the breath. Similarly, hatha yoga tells us that by becoming aware of and accessing the breath consciously in these ways we can also access directly into our **psycho-neurology**, the biopsychic pathways, nadis, matrices, energy cysts, and cellular and energetic imprints which hold the samskaras in place, thus breaking them up, breaking up past karma, kleshas, and vrttis (root desires).

Thus the various pranayama exercises of exploring the energetic processes of inhalation, exhalation, and holding of breath especially in Gitananda Rishiculture Yoga were given to Sadakas in order to achieve this awareness, observe this process, and thus eventually achieve purity of body, mind and emotions followed by karmic purification to attain liberation (from karma and vrtti). The goal is not the control of the breath. Our goal is to inculcate the awareness of the subtle and eternal operations of prana shakti or kundalini shakti.

In many practices of hatha yoga, laya yoga, and prana vidya, control of the normal flow of the breath are given in order to both develop awareness and oneness. The Second aim is to disrupt old mental patterns (vrttis) and karma fructifying the previous dormant or energy to spiritual evolution. In these innumerable pranayama practices one has the opportunity to investigate many types of breathing patterns upon on our energy field and thus becoming aware of the breath processes (vicchedah), then one becomes more aware and integrated with Vital Prana.

"Normal" subconscious habitual breathing is thus called karmic breathing, while pranayama practice not only breaks up old karma, but burns it up to make the practitioner free of karmic bondage. Here various pranayama practices using the breath can be used for healing, and propelling the practitioner beyond their past conditioning and karma altogether. Just simple breath awareness helps us to free the dissipations of the 'monkey-like' mind (vikalpa) and concentrates the chi-prana. In Rishiculture tradition pranayama practices go deeper and work faster combining, pranayama, pratyhara, dharana, mudra, and asana as one integrated practice.

In simple pranayama like sukha-pranayama or the vibhhaga pranayama we can simply notice the changing qualities of breath according to how the mind becomes distracted or focused. We bring our awareness to the breath and refine and extend it if it has become coarse or restricted. After practice this relationship between the empty and quiet mind and the breath becomes harmonious and a doorway opens into the operations of the cit-prana and the operations of the mind. Then eventually the origin of mind, the Infinite Mind, or simply the Natural Unconditioned Mind is revealed through at first the very simple method of learning how to observe the breath and how it changes. Then one learns how to balance and direct the cit-prana, the mind, and the breath all at once.

Pranayama brings us into awareness of the polar opposites, the expansion and the contraction of the divine pulsation of siva/shakti (spanda), the movement of spirit as it inspires, and eternal dance of love through the expiratory medium of the living temple.

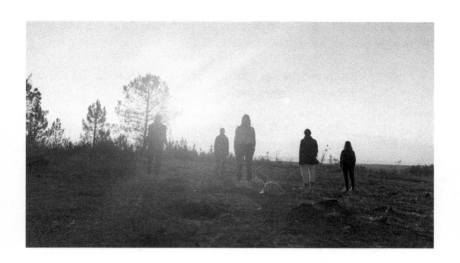

Basic Requirements for Good Pranayama

First if you have any of the breathing problems related to shallow breathing that should be corrected. Then the environmental conditions should be also considered to be free from dust or a damp atmosphere. Proper sectional breathing should be practiced. Your mat should be thin and firm, like a rubber-foam pad. A thick mattress stuffed with the cotton and other softeners tends to catch the dust, and germs detrimental to correct breathing.

Your room should be regularly cleaned. Never allow the dirt to accumulate on the walls, corners, and other cloths you are using. Bed covers and other cloths should be of cotton.

Use of powders, fumes, scents, essences, body lotions etc should be avoided and especially in case you have any allergic problems. You may be allergic to the soap, tooth powder, or the facial creams, be aware and avoid the harmful things.

The preparation should be done properly before starting the pranayama or the hatha yoga practice, ideal conditions are:

- Comb and tie up your hair properly. Loose hair may create problems in complete breathing.

- Clean your body before the practice by having a light warm bath. Please never take too hot or too cool bath before the hatha yoga practice.

- Clean, loose comfortable clothes should be worn if possible. Tight clothes, jewellery, belts, etc should be avoided.

- After the yoga practice a cool shower should be taken. This will strengthens the body tolerance power to cold air and water. Although this will depend on where you live in the world!

- Keep your mat properly folded and covered with the cotton cloths to avoid the damp and dust.

- Your area of practising yoga should be well-ventilated with plenty of fresh air.

- Do all the practice at least after three hours of eating food. All practices should be done with an empty stomach. A light tea, lemon or limewater can be taken. Avoid all mucus producing foods. If there is any desire to empty the bowel or bladder, do so, as a priority.

Prana, Thoughts and Emotions

Try to remember the situation when you are very happy and cheerful; how do you feel about your body and about your self at that time? You feel very light, energetic, and willing to do everything at that moment. What is behind all this?

Now remember the situation when you are sad, unhappy and in bad mood; how do you feel about your body and yourself? You feel very heavy, tired, exhausted, lack of interest and will. What is behind all this?

As we have discussed, all of our physical, mental and emotional process are carried on through the energy of prana. So our mental and emotional states directly affect the levels of prana in us. All the negative thoughts, stress and negative emotions blocks the refinement of prana and flow of the prana in the naris (also known as nadis, energy channels in the body). They consume a high amount of the prana because the negative thoughts create the body reactions of an 'emergency state'. Our autonomic nervous system and the endocrine nervous system have to prepare for the fight-flight response. This consumes a lot of prana and preparation for nothing. So be careful about what you think and feel.

Patanjali describes that in all the adverse mental and emotional processes use the opposite thought or the emotion to get rid of the negativity (prati-paksha-bhavanam).

It is also stated in the Upanishadas that your prana goes where your awareness goes. So the more distracted your thoughts and emotions are, the more your prana is scattered or poor. Paradoxically, the more refined your awareness is the greater your power to manifest your thoughts.

In the Bhagavad-Gita Lord Krishna states that the mind is the vehicle of prana. Thus your awareness goes where your thought goes. Your mind goes where your awareness goes and there goes the prana. Thus the mind or the thoughts and emotions need the prana or the consciousness to travel in and out. Those who do mental work at the end of the day feel more tired in comparison to the person doing only physical work, why? Our mental and emotional processes consume more prana than the physical process. So be careful and be aware of what you think and what you feel, develop your awareness of the mental and emotional processes.

Prana- Philosophical Aspect

According to Indian schools of philosophies, i.e. Upanishads, Samkhya, Advaita, etc., the body is divided in two parts – the gross physical body (sthul sarira) and the subtle body (linga sarira), both include five Pranas, the mind (mental body), the intellectual (buddhi) and the self-sense (ahankara). The gross physical body is composed of five elements. According to Nyaya philosophy the body is the vehicle of action for the self. The mind along with all sense organs is found to operate only within the human body. All feelings of pleasure and pain in the body are due the destiny (karma). Balanced functioning of sympathetic and parasympathetic parts of the nervous system is necessary for the harmony in all these, described above.

The Indian yogis described the energy of Prana, as the vital energy essential for a living being. According to some of the six Indian philosophies "Prana is a subtle life-force". Sometimes it is represented as an electromagnetic force or bioelectric force in the body, but these cannot exactly be described as the Prana, though these are similar to the Prana. The term Prana is more appropriate to describe the Prana as the vital life force.

Prana sustains and supports this body. All the bodily activities are dependent of the pranic energy. According to Indian Yoga, "When the Queen bee goes up all the Bees go up, and as the Queen Bee settles down all the Bees settle down, when so, speech, mind, sense are balanced when the energy of Prana is balanced in human body.

According to the six schools of Indian philosophies, everything in this universe is composed of cosmic energy, Prana. In various schools, like Vedic, Samkhya, Jain etc., the Prana is classified in five categories, which flow in various parts of the body and regulates their concerned functions. In upanishadas and other tantric yogic texts five up-pranas are also stated and detailed.

Pancha Vayus

Pancha Vayus

Vayu	Body Region	Movement	Area Between	Function
1. Prana	heart region	Inward and Rising Upward	larynx and diaphragm	breathing, food and liquid swallowing
2. Apana	lower regions	Outward and Downward	Navel and perineum	Elimination of urine, faeces, gas, wind, sexual fluids, menstrual blood, and the fetus at the time of birth
3. Samana	Digestive area	Lateral Flow	Diaphragm and navel	All digestive functions and also the heating and cooling of the body
4. Udana	Peripheral parts	Spiraling Upward	Above the larynx and also the arms	Brain and all sensory receptors- eyes, ears, nose, tongue and skin are governed as well as three organs of action- speech, hands and feet
5. Vyana	All-pervasive	All directions	Whole body	Reserve force for all four and maintenance of their depletion, regulation of physical movements

Pancha Upa-Prana Vayus

Upa-prana	Function
Naga	Belching, vomiting or spitting
Korma	Flickering of the eyes
Krikariya	Sneezing
Devadatta	Yawning
Dhananjaya	Physical warmth and will remain in the body for some time even after death

For controlling the senses, thoughts and emotions, it is not enough to acknowledge the anatomy and physiology of the human body, but also to be familiar with the flow of Prana. Hence for spiritual masteries, it is necessary to perceive the body as a whole. The process of body perception is the process of regulation of the prana in the body and development of detachment with that of the outer world and attachment with the internal world. Hence it is the process of introversion and awakening of spiritualism.

Naris and Pranayama

The yoga science describes 72000 nadis; important among these are six, Ida, pingla, sushumna, brahmani, chitrani and vijnana. Most important are pingla (surya), which flow through right nostril; ida (Chandra), which flow through left nostril; sushumna (central) that is a movement when both nostrils flow freely without any obstruction.

Nari	Body Part
1. Ida Nari-	Left Side of Body
2. Pingala Nari	Right side of body
3. Shusumna Nari	Middle of body
4. Gandhari	left eye
5. Hastajiva	right eye
6. Pusha	right ear
7. Yashasavini	left ear
8. Alambusa	Facial region
9. Kuhu	Genitals
10. Shakini	Perineum

All these major nadis originate at the base of spine and travel upwards. The sushumna nadi is centrally located and travel along the spinal cord. At the level of larynx it divides into an anterior portion and a posterior portion, both of which terminate in the brahmarandra, or in the cavity of Brahma. The ida and pingla also travel upwards along the spinal column, but they criss-cross the sushumna, before terminating in the left and right nostrils.

The junctions of the ida, the pingla, and the sushumna are known as charkas or wheels. There are seven principle chakras according to various Indian schools of yoga. These are: -

1. The muladhara chakra, (at the base of spine at the level of pelvic plexus).
2. The swadhishthana chakra (at the level of hypo gastric plexus).
3. The manipura chakra (at the level of solar plexus).
4. Anahata chakra (at the level of cardiac plexus).
5. The vishuddhia chakra (at the level of pharyngeal plexus).
6. The ajna chakra (at the level of the nasoscilliary plexus).
7. The sahasrara chakra (at the top of head).

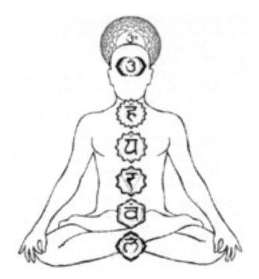

A fraction of the total energy of prana is used in dynamic and creative aspect; the major part of it is being in a potential, or seed state. The stored up energy is known as kundalini in manuals of yoga, the symbolic representation of which is that of a sleeping serpent rolled up in the muladhara charka, at the base of the spine. In the average individual there is flow of prana through the Ida and the pingla, but not through the sushumna, the nadi being blocked at the base of the spinal column.

LOCATION OF THE CHAKRAS

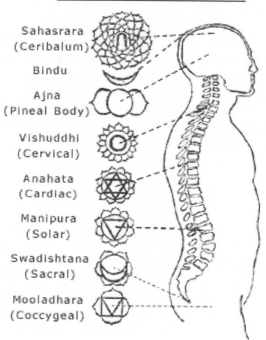

Sahasrara
(Ceribalum)

Bindu

Ajna
(Pineal Body)

Vishuddhi
(Cervical)

Anahata
(Cardiac)

Manipura
(Solar)

Swadishtana
(Sacral)

Mooladhara
(Coccygeal)

Pranayama is aimed to balance the ida and pingala nari to allow the free flow of the prana in the sushumna nari to attain the unity or the oneness with the supreme self. Pranayama opens all the blockages created because of our unhealthy life style and bad karmas. Pranayama refines and purifies the gross prana to the subtle and pure chitta-prana which enables us to feel the joy of oneness or samadhi the highest stage of yoga. This purification is a must for all the yogic seekers if you really want to grow on the path of yogic evolution. You have to purify your body, thoughts, emotions, karmas, and then gross prana to the subtle prana.

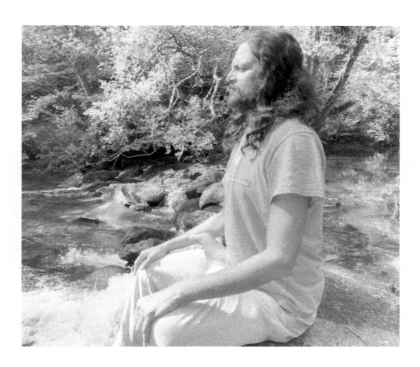

Pratyahara- Sensory Withdrawal.

Ahara means food for the body, as well as thoughts, experiences and information for our mind through the sensory organs. Pratya means reversing or opposing. Pratyahara is the fifth limb of Ashtanga or Raja Yoga which means "withdrawing the mind away from the objects of senses".

Many may translate Pratyahara as control of the sense organs. However, closing your eyes or ears, or desensitising the sense organs, is not the practice of Pratyahara. Pratyahara is focusing our mind, not letting it wildly wander so it does not get distracted by sensory information.

Our sense organs (Indriyas) are responsible for receiving all the information and passing it to our brain through the nerve pathways or neurons. Our brain and mind analyses this information and create the experience of liking or disliking (raga-dvesha), wanting or not wanting (iccha-anichha), and pain or pleasure (sukha-dukha). Separating our senses from the objects of senses is known as Asamprayoga. Our sensory information is one of the causes of the modifications or whirlpools of our mind known as chitta-vrittis. Due to our innate nature our senses and mind are active and outgoing. Pratyahara is the process used to reverse this outward movement of the mind and senses in order to develop the ability to focus our mind inward, which leads us to practice and master Samayoga (dharna, dhyana and samadhi).

In Sanskrit, the senses are known as Indriyas, or the instruments of Indra, the lord of heaven. In Yoga they represent the instruments of pain and pleasure experience and are seen as divine instruments in the microcosm of the body. The spiritual tradition recognises 10 senses, namely five organs of action (karmendriyas) and five organs of cognition (jnanendriyas). The mind is described as the Indra, or their master. Yogic traditions also include the mind, intellect and ahamkara (manas, buddhi and ego) as subtle sense organs too which makes it 13 senses.

The Jnanendriyas are:

Chaksu – the eyes

Srotra, or Karna – the ears

Ghrana, or Nasagra – the nose

Rasana or Jivya – the tongue

Tvacha – the skin (tvacha).

The karmendiryas are:

Pani or Hasta – the hands

Pada – the feet or legs

Vak – the speech or vocal cord

Payu -the anus or excretory organs

Upasta – the sexual organs

According to the Bhagavad Gita, "the mind or the manas is the controller of the sense organs. Our senses are functioning or acting under the instructions and intentions of mind".

Patanjali in the Yoga Sutras mentions that successful practice of pratyahara enables the sadhaka to master their mind, and the operating fields of the mind, preparing them for the higher three limbs of ashtanga yoga.

Dharana – Concentration Practice

Dharana is to focus our wandering mind on a single point or object of concentration. This is the inner practice of gazing our mind on an object, image, thought, mantra and mandala for a long period of time. The goal of dharana is to gradually develop the single-pointed focus of our mind and stabilise it.

Even though it is known that our mind is fickle and always actively busy in chitta-vrittis or whirlpools of the mind, Patanjali mentions that "our mind holds the ability to focus on a single point." The Yoga scriptures teach us that by withdrawing our mind from the outer world we can experience an abundance of inner peace and unconditional joy. By keeping the mind focused on our True Nature or Inner Self (atman), and the practice of Dharana is the effort needed to attain or master that state of oneness or meditation.

Dharana is continuously, with effort, drawing our mind again and again back to our concentration or focus point and not letting the mind wander around freely.

Krishna in the Bhagavad Gita mentions that "a sadhaka should sit straight in a comfortable Asana, focus the mind at the tip of nose and witness the incoming and outgoing breath as a Dharna." He further mentions that every time you find your mind wandering around, gently try to bring your mind back to the breath awareness and keep repeating this to master your mind. This is one typical example of Dharana or concentration practice.

Tantric scriptures describe around 118 dharana or concentration techniques.

Dhyana – Meditation

To begin with remember Dhyana is not the practice, but a fruit of Dharana or concentration practice. So, if Dharana is your effort to focus on a single point, when the mind is fully absorbed or becomes one with the point of focus it is known as the state of Dhyana or meditation. Dhyana is total absorption of the mind on the focus point, interest, thought, mantra or inclination (abhimata).

Ammaji Meenakshi Devi mentions that "Dharana is to focus our mind more and more on less and less, while Dhyana is absorption of our mind in that ultimate focus point itself."

Dhyana is the state of total mindfulness where your body, senses, mind, awareness, thoughts and feelings become one. It is the state where you are free from judgements or the duality of pain-pleasure (dukkha-sukha), liking-disliking (raga-dvesha) etc.

Dhyana can be experienced passively by being a mere observer or witness without interfering with the activities of the mind, or you may experience it by an active process of channelling the mind, thoughts and energy in a particular direction.

Maharishi Patanjali mentions that "regular meditation practice eliminates the afflictions (kleshas) of the mind." He further mentions that "the fruits or siddhis (spiritual masteries) of dhyana or meditation do not produce karmic consequences or fruits."

How to Meditate

Human beings are moving towards spiritual teachings in search of mental peace. They try to feel calm and relaxed by using the medicine of spiritual teachings.

Like a drug addiction, some 'spiritual' teachings are also one type of addiction. Sometimes this may be so deep that it may cause family disputes.

Distance is developed between husband and wife. This distance may be so long that it may result in the breaking of relations.

Spirituality always binds the person with the person. That is not spirituality, which cause disputes in us. Can you call it spirituality that forms a wall between two?

Tension cannot be released by the action based meditation techniques and the ways of addiction. The action-based means may result in forgetting the tension for some time but this could not make one free from the stress.

Tension is released by meditation, but people have changed the picture of meditation in to pictures of actions. In the classes of meditation various activities are introduced in the name of meditation.

Reactions cannot be changed by the reactions. Reactions can be changed by inaction. Meditation is not action but meditation is inaction.

Meenakshi Devi Bhavanani often said during her satsanga (at Ananda Ashram, Puducherry, India) that "meditation is concentrating more and more on less and less, finally this becomes nothing or one-ness with dharana, and that merging in the self is called meditation, one needs to be purified to tolerate this stage of meditation". One should be physically stable and balanced, mentally and emotionally pure and calm. The brain should be healthy to perceive the mind and emotions. The naris should be purified for free flow of the prana from the lower charkas to the higher. This could be attained through the practices of asanas, Pranayama, and cleansing techniques.

We are prisoners of the sense organs and have to work in the outer world, so sense control through pratyahara should be perfected. Even **Dr. Swami Gitananda Giri** states that "the perfection of yamas and niyamas is the pre-condition to grow on the yogic path and this is compulsory for one and all".

Speech and listening also influences your progress in the path of meditation. Condition your mind in such a way that you speak and listen to things promoting you towards enlightenment. Do not waste time in gossiping, and in agitating thoughts and activities. The Mind is led to dullness by regular opposition of the light of Viveka. This can be enlightened by the practice of reflection, concentration and spiritual enquiry.

One can attain relaxation and stillness of body and mind through meditation. How do we meditate? When you come to this point we need to understand that meditation is **'not doing'**, or keeping our mind busy in structured practices or full of imaginative visualisations. However, our mind is so conditioned with our experiences, language, culture etc... therefore we always misunderstand the actual meaning of meditation. Meditation is going beyond all our 'doings' i.e. Physical, mental and imaginative processes. For this level to be reached, one must practise and repeat many of the breathing and structured relaxation techniques in order to break our conditioning.

To attain this world we have to consider the body and mind. We cannot perform the worldly activities without means of actions. The word and action is necessary to be with this physical world. But if you want to go beyond this world than one should be free from word and action. The body travels to action and mind up to the words. We trained the body for activities and taught words to the mind.

At the time of the body's birth it was unaware of the action. The brain possesses no words. The brain was empty. In whichever environment the bodies grow, the brain learned the language of the concerned area. The child learns from family members. We teach her/him to do something with her/his hands etc.

The senses are trained like this as s/he grows. The senses have the natural powers to do the actions. The brain also has an inborn ability to learn words. Our nature is inborn 'animal like' and it will remain so unless we learn higher aspects in this or the next life...

In the field of duties, the body and mind are important; word and action are valuable. But we have to go to the field of meditation. This is not the field of body and mind but it is the field of conscious, which is out of the reach of body and mind.

The body is visible and soul is invisible. The world is visible and the supreme soul is invisible. Now you want to say that we always try to visualize but cannot perceive it. The body has the ability to do only activities.

When the individual feels tired after actions, the energy is consumed the activities are stopped and relaxed. The power of perception of each sense organ has limitations. After a limit all activities are stopped.

It is also true that the brain have many unlimited abilities. The bird of the mind can fly in the space of imagination. But each bird has its limitations. If it will fly away from its limits then it is going to fall down. If the vehicle of the mind runs faster than the limits, it may also be damaged. The excessive use of the mind or the excessive weight of the words on the mind results in the mental imbalances which manifest in physical problems.

To gain this success we have to learn to meditate. The balance should be established between the action and word. The music to balance the body and mind is to be learned.

To meditate we consider the body and mind to catch the thread of action and word. The use of word and action is useful for the travelling of the external physical world; we can go on the steps of physical development. The help of action and word should be left to travel the internal world. If we try to enter the internal world along with the thread of action and world, there will be an opposing conflict.

The body and mind are god-gifted vehicles. The travelling of humanity and service in the nature of God is to be started by using these vehicles. Vehicles (bodies) are very important to go outside the home and to come back to the door of your home. Do you enter in your personal room with your vehicle? You leave your vehicle at your home's gate and then enter into your home.

When the senses begin to rest inward, rather than being distracted outwardly, then it means the vehicle returns back to home from the visit. Now you have to leave the vehicle and go for the rest in your personal room for the deep rest. Your personal room is full of the essence of peace. There is joy everywhere in that room, it is termed supreme soul. It is always present there. This stage is attained by consciousness/awareness. But our awareness learned the travelling in the visible world along with the body and mind.

Sadguru taught that the practice of rest in self-room is inaction meditation, or not doing, going beyond doing. The vehicle returns back home. Fatigue of body and mind is released. Tension is also released. Awareness is merged in self. Where the awareness always meets with the psyche, there is wordless rest.

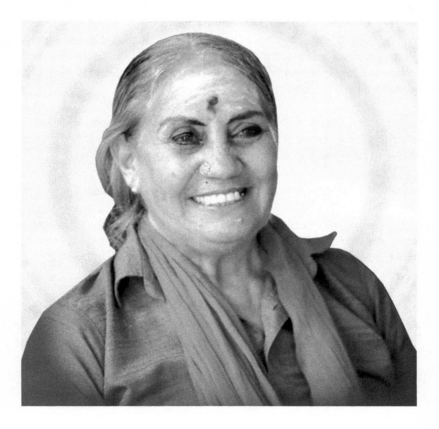

Samadhi – Union, Oneness, Self-Realisation

Samadhi is a Sanskrita term (combination of 'Sama means equal, one, or union' and 'adhi means eternal or prior, ever existing') which means 'union with the real self' or 'total absorption in the Self or Purusha'. Samadhi is the ultimate goal and fruit of Yoga Sadhana. This is the state where the Sadhaka enters after a prolonged, gradual and disciplined Yoga Sadhana.

According to Paramahansa Yogananda, "Samadhi is a soundless state of breathlessness." The word Samadhi can be broken down as sam, "together" or "integrated"; ā, "towards"; dhā, "to get, to hold": Samadhi therefore translates as "to acquire integration or wholeness, or truth; a blissful super consciousness state in which a yogi perceives the identity of the individualised Soul and Cosmic Spirit."

Most of our lives are caught up in mundane physical, mental and emotional activities, which are the seed cause of our identification with Samsara, or the material world subject to change, birth and death. This takes us away from our true self and most of us see the body, birth or our material existence as the Real Self. Seeing the body as the Self is Ajnana or ignorance in Yogic Terms.

As a Yoga Sadhaka we begin to realise the 'we are not the body'. Here we see the Self and the Divine Self (Atma-Parmatma, Jiva-Iswara) as two separate identities - this is known as Dvaita or duality. In Samadhi we experience the oneness of the Self with the Supreme Self, which is known as Advaita or Non-duality. Samadhi is the absolute absorption of the self in the supreme self, from where the Jiva attains liberation from the worldly suffering (Samsara-Vedana) and attains absolute bliss known as Sat-Chit-Ananda.

Samadhi is also understood as the awakening of the self from the state of ignorance or sleep (not knowing the true identity of the Self) known as Atma-Jnana. Here only the witnessing awareness of the Self or Purusha remains awakened – this is known as Sakshi Bhava, free from any separateness or otherness. According to Maharishi Patanjali, here a Sadhaka experiences the absolute wisdom as taught in the Scriptures or Shastras by Great Yogis and Rishis.

Patanjali mentions various levels of Samadhi as follows:

· Savikalpa, or Samprajnata – In this state of Samadhi there is still awareness of the object of focus or concentration.

· Nirvikalpa, or Asamprajnata – In this state of Samadhi, the Sadhaka is free from identification with the object of focus and is fully absorbed in the manas or consciousness.

· Sabija Samadhi – In this state of Samadhi the seeds of Karma and samaskaras are still there.

· Nirbija Samadhi – In this Samadhi, one becomes absolutely free from any form of the seeds of Karma, samaskara, object and its identifications.

Yoga is To Live in Equanimity (Yoga Samatva)

Samatva is one of the commonly known as a very important practice in Yogic, Vedic and Vedantic traditions. It means living and maintaining the state of equanimity, equality, indifference or uniformity in all the ups and downs of our life. The term Samatva comes from the Sanskrit root, sama, which means "equal."

Lord Krishna in Bhagavat Gita explains Arjuna to master and live in balanced, calm, and even-mindedness. He says that "you all your duties with offering them to me, divine cause and let go the desires and attachment towards fruits or outcome". He says a Yogi should remain calm and mindful in adverse and favourable situations.

It can also be practised by maintaining body and mind equanimity. Our body and mind respond, react or act to each others state of being. If we are not feeling happy, our body feels stress too. Similarly if our body in pain, our mind feels sad too. This is also a state of awareness where our body and mind are doing the same thing. If you are going for a walk, you are walking fully conscious and not letting your mind wander around in other activities.

In mastering this state of equality, we become free from transitory states of duality like – like-dislike, pain-pleasure, good-bad, and life-death. , a person is said to have overcome the transitory conditions of birth and death. Here you do everything as it needs to be done by you or it is your duty, not because you like or not like it.

Lord Krishna in Bhagavat Gita says that success and failure should be treated alike. In following this you will become be indifference to such ups and downs, success and failure and thus, attains liberated from them. He further says that one who practises equanimity, sees all beings in the same way, regardless of their outward appearance, cast, colour, or status because everyone has the same potential and divine Self or Atman.

Samatva can be mastered through Karma Yoga, Hatha Yoga and Jnana Yoga practices as they bring tranquility and stability.

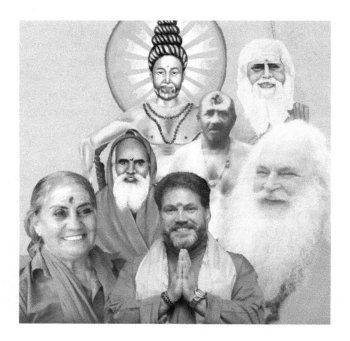

Be Aware to avoid the Miseries Yet to Come

Yoga advocates that we should try to live in harmony with our true nature, be in the moment here and now, take responsibility for everything that we do or every choice we make. This allows us to be in tune with our true nature.

We all have a gut instinct or gut feeling. It always tells us what is to be done and what is to be avoided. Many adverse situations can be avoided by following our heart and inner self. As Arjuna asks Krishna, why do we do immoral, unhealthy or wrong things. Krishna explains that it is because of our desires, asmita or I-ness and ahamkara that leads us in doing many things that even we wouldn't approve of ourselves. When desire takes our viveka or discriminative mind, we want to fulfil them at any cost. When we cant fulfil them, it leads to anger, irritation, and discontentment, which further causes physical, mental and emotional imbalance and turmoil.

Swamiji Dr Gitananda Giri ji mentions that "health and happiness are our birth rights." But we all need to claim it and maintain it in our day to day life. We cant take our health and well-being for granted. We need to avoid all that is causing discomfort, pain or stress to our body-mind health. We need to avoid all the junk food, avoid any food that we are allergic to. We need to make sure that we ignore our day to day physical practice to keep our body health, fit and strong. This is what Patanjali says here- "take responsibility, be aware and listen your heart, to avoid many problems yet to come".

We can also avoid many adverse situations in our day to day life and interactions to prevent conflicts. Most people are quite fragile and volatile these days. If we can hold ourselves back and give a bit of space in our relations and adverse situations for a little while, we find much better clarity for our thoughts, and emotions. We are in the middle of crisis or conflict, we tend to lose our reasoning, intellect and tend to make choices or actions under the volcano of anger, frustration or guilt. If you can allow some space and try to evaluate the events and situations without being victim to them, you will find much better and calmer ways to deal with the same situation or issue.

Yoga – Uniting the Self and Supreme Self

Yoga is the process of taking us back to our un-distracted true nature. Yoga is the process of being one with self and the supreme self. Yoga is aimed to refine and purify all our mental, emotional and karmic bondages.

The Yoga-Sutras define that stage of mental and emotional destruction as not natural but modified. These modifications and afflictions are called chitta-vrttis. The state, called chitta-vrtti, is mankind's general (but not inborn) condition. It is a distorted and impaired state of disturbed or agitated (vrtti) consciousness (chitta). It is like sun rays passing through coloured glass.
Vrttis attach to the chitta producing vrtti-chitta; that is, resulting in various thought patterns, emotions, feelings, destruction, and agitation. This separates self from its true nature and results in our dualistic nature.

Swami Vivekananda says that **"The chitta, by its own nature, is endowed with all knowledge. It is made of sattva particles, but is covered by rajas and tamas particles; and by pranayama this covering is removed."** (page 181 Raja Yoga)

Yoga can be described as a "tool" of deprogramming this negative conditioning - liberating the individual's modified consciousness from the conditioned consciousness of "non-reality" back into this Original, Natural, and Unmodified state of "Reality".

Thus yoga is a step by step approach by which confused, lonely, destructed, bounded consciousness can be reunited, harmonized, and integrated with its true nature and the Sadhaka can attain intimate sense of belonging in the world, of profound well being, contentment, fulfilment, peace, and joy.
Yoga is aimed to bring us into samadhi (the experience of transpersonal and non-dual union/absorption). Yoga is to attain self- realization called nirbija samadhi (samadhi without seed), wherein even the seeds of future vrttis have become eliminated and dissolved (nirodha) in the state of chitta-vrtti-nirodha.

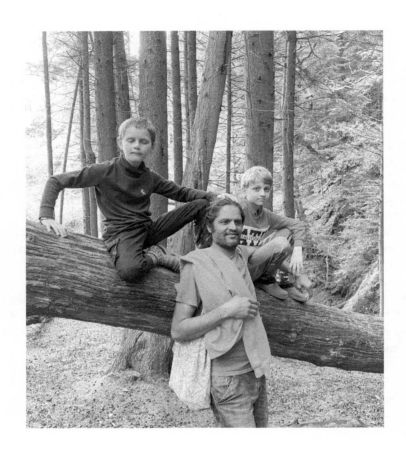

Yoga: The Ideal Way Of Life

Yogacharya Dr Ananda Balayogi Bhavanani

Chairman: International Centre for Yoga Education and Research (ICYER), Ananda Ashram, Pondicherry, India. www.icyer.com and www.rishiculture.org

INTRODUCTION:

Yoga is gradually being welcomed into modern health care systems as an understanding of its multifarious benefits is gaining ground worldwide. In our haste to have it accepted into the mainstream medicare, we must not however forget that Yoga is first and foremost a spiritual science for the integrated, holistic development of the physical, mental and spiritual aspects of our being. Though the recent advancements in the field of research have given evidence that Yoga helps normalize human physiological and psychological functioning more importantly the practice of Yoga as a way of life is calming and provides a rare opportunity in our chaotic lives to leave the madness of the outside world behind and attain an inner peace by helping us to focus inwards.

The World health organisation defines health as "The state of complete physical, mental and social wellbeing and not merely absence of disease or infirmity". The Yogic way of living is a vital tool that helps attain that 'state' of health. We must not forget that it is more important to have both a sense of "being" healthy as well as "feeling" healthy. Hence, the qualitative aspect of health, the spiritual nature of the human life is rightly considered more important in Yoga and other Indian systems of traditional medicine.

The Bhagavad Gita defines Yoga as equanimity at all levels which may also be taken as the perfect state of health where there is physical homeostasis and mental equanimity giving rise to a healthy harmony between the body and mind. The Hatha Yoga Pradipika, also states that "Yoga improves the health of all alike and wards off diseases of one who tirelessly practices Yoga whether they are young, old, decrepit, diseased or weak, provided they abide to the rules and regulations properly".

THE ORIGINAL MIND BODY MEDICINE:

Yoga is the original mind body medicine and is one of the greatest treasures of the unique Indian cultural heritage. As both an art and science it has a lot to offer humankind in terms of an understanding of both the human mind as well as all aspects of our multilayered existence. Yoga treats man as a multi layered, conscious being, possessing three bodies (sthula, sukshma and kaarana sharira) and being enveloped in a five layered (pancha kosha) of existence.

This ancient science of mind control as codified by Maharishi Patanjali more than 2500 years ago helps us to understand our mental processes as well as the cause - effect relations of a multitude of problems facing modern man. Modern man is the victim of stress and stress related disorders that threaten to disrupt his life totally. Yoga offers a way out of this 'whirlpool of stress' and is a wholistic solution to stress.

Yogic lifestyle, Yogic diet, Yogic attitudes and various Yogic practices help man to strengthen himself and develop positive health thus enabling him to withstand stress better. This Yogic "health insurance" is achieved by normalizing the perception of stress, optimizing the reaction to it and by releasing the pent up stress effectively through various Yogic practices. Yoga is a wholistic and integral science of life dealing with physical, mental, emotional and spiritual health of the individual and society.

A PERSONAL EVOLUTIONARY JOURNEY

Yoga is a continuous process. The whole problem with something being goal-oriented is that people think that the goal is something to be reached at the end of the journey, but it is the journey itself that is important. This entire yogic process is not what you learn and not what you achieve. Yoga is something that you "live" until your last breath, and even that last breath should be completed with awareness. You should go with the satisfaction of knowing that you have done your best. Yoga is a continuous process. It is a journey and the goal is the journey itself.

Yoga is getting to know what your body can and cannot do. Yoga is watching the breath, slowing down the breath and discovering that you can have a wonderful control over your emotions when slowing down the breath, because breath is the seat of our emotions. Yoga is not about the number of Yoga practices we do nor is it about how many times or how long we do them. It is all about how we live our life in tune with Dharma.

This is all about our evolutionary journey from the lower animal states of being to the highest divine states of being that has been beautifully described by the Sufi Saint Rumi hundreds of years ago. Rumi declared in ecstasy, "I died as a mineral to become a plant, I died as a plant to become an animal, I died as an animal to become a man, I died as a man to become an angel, I died as an angel to become a God. When was I ever the less by dying"?

Yoga is life and everything we do is Yoga. Yoga is in every second of life, Yoga is in every action you do and in every thought you have and in every emotion that you feel. For modern man in a modern setting, I feel more than anything else that Yoga is skill in action. Whatever you do, you should do with the attitude that it is to be done to the best of your ability and with total effort. I think that to have action that is skilful and yet not motivated by any desire is a model concept for modern man. I see Yoga, in its modern context, as skilful action without desire or concern about the fruits of our actions.

YOGA AND HEALTH :

Yoga understands health and well being as a dynamic continuum of human nature and not a mere 'state' to be attained and maintained. The lowest point on the continuum with the lowest speed of vibration is that of death whereas the highest point with the highest vibration is that of immortality. In between these two extremes lie the states of normal health and disease. For many, their state of health is defined as that 'state' in which they are able to function without hindrance whereas in reality, health is part of our evolutionary process towards Divinity. The lowest point on the dynamic health continuum with lowest speed of vibration may be equated with lowest forms of life and mineral matter while the highest point with highest speed of vibration may be equated with Divinity.

The Yogic concept of health and disease enables us to understand that the cause of physical disorder sprouts from the higher levels of the mind and beyond. Adhi – the disturbed mind is the cause and vyadhi - the disease is the effect manifested in the physical body. Maharishi Patanjali mentions "vyadhi" as a hindrance to the complete integration of the individual personality. He doesn't directly refer to the treatment of particular diseases as his approach is more holistic and expanded rather than analytical and limited. Patanjali prefers to 'integrate' rather than deal exclusively with individual symptoms of dis-integration. The diseases are merely gross symptoms that accompany disturbances of the mind called vikshepa which appear as duhkha (misery or pain), daurmanasya (dejection), angamejayatva (tremors) and svasaprasvasa, (disturbances in breathing). Through the Yoga life, one can control these disturbances before they become powerful enough to cause breakdown. The two-pronged attack advised by Patanjali is holistic: yama-niyama on the psychological side and asana-pranayama on the physical.

DEALING WITH OMNIPRESENT STRESS

Thousands of years ago, Yogeshwar Krishna in the Bhagavad Gita (often referred to as the bible of Yoga) taught us about the Yogic patho–psychology of stress and how through our attraction to the worldly sensory objects we cause our own destruction. These potent ancient teachings hold true even in today's world. In chapter Two (Samkhya Yoga), the pattern of behaviour (stress response) is given that ultimately leads to the destruction of man. In verse 62 Lord Krishna says,

Bhavanani AB. Yoga: The ideal way of life. Yoga Mimamsa 2013; 44(4): 314-25.

"Brooding on the objects of the senses, man develops attachment to them; from attachment (sanga or chanuraaga) comes desire (kama) and from unfulfilled desire, anger (krodha) sprouts forth." Verse 63 tells us, "From anger proceeds delusion (moha); from delusion, confused memory (smriti vibramah); from confused memory the ruin of reason and due to the ruin of reason (buddhi naaso) he perishes." In the very next verse (64), he also gives us a clue to equanimity of mind (samatvam) and how to become a person settled in that equanimity (stitha prajna) who is not affected by the opposites (dwandwa). He says, "but the disciplined yogi, moving amongst the sensory objects with all senses under control and free from attraction (raaga) and aversion (dwesha), gains in tranquillity."

According to Maharishi Patanjali, most of our problems stem from the five psycho- physiological afflictions (pancha klesha) that are inborn in each and every human being. These pancha klesha are ignorance (avidya), egoism (asmita) and our sense of needing to survive at any cost (abinivesha) as well as the attraction (raaga) to external objects and the repulsion (dwesha) to them. Ignorance (avidya) is usually the start of most problems along with the ego (asmita). Our sense of needing to survive at any cost (abinivesha) compounds it further. Both attraction (raaga) to external objects and the repulsion (dwesha) to them need to be destroyed in order to attain tranquillity as well as equanimity of emotions and the mind. Maharishi Patanjali further states that the practice of Kriya

Yoga (Yoga of mental purification) consisting of tapa (disciplined effort), svadhyaya (self analysis) and ishwara pranidhana (surrender to the Divine will) is the means to destroy these five mental afflictions and attain to the state of samadhi or oneness with the supreme self or the Divine.

The regular practice of yogasana, kriya, mudra, bandha and pranayama helps to recondition the physical (annamaya kosha) and energy (pranamaya kosha) bodies. The practice of pratyahara, dharana and dhyana techniques helps to recondition the mind body (manomaya kosha) apparatus. All of these Yogic practices help to foster a greater mind-emotions-body understanding and bring about the union and harmony of body, emotions and mind. This righteous (right-use-ness) union is Yoga in its truest sense.

Yoga helps us to take the right attitude towards our problems and thus tackle them in an effective manner. "To have the will (iccha shakti) to change (kriya shakti) that which can be changed, the strength to accept that which can not he changed, and the wisdom (jnana shakti) to know the difference" is the attitude that needs to the cultivated. An attitude of letting go of the worries, the problems and a greater understanding of our mental process helps to create a harmony in our body, and mind whose disharmony is the main cause of 'aadi – vyadhi' or psychosomatic disorders.

PRODUCING POSITIVE HEALTH AND WELL BEING

According to Swami Kuvalayananda, founder of Kaivalyadhama positive health does not mean mere freedom from disease but is a jubilant and energetic way of living and feeling that is the peak state of well being at all levels – physical, mental, emotional, social and spiritual. He says that one of the aims of Yoga is to encourage positive hygiene and health through development of inner natural powers of body and mind. In doing so, Yoga gives special attention to various eliminative processes and reconditions inherent powers of adaptation and adjustment of body and mind. Thus, the

development of positive powers of adaptation and adjustment, inherent to the internal environment of man, helps him enjoy positive health and not just mere freedom from disease. He emphasizes that Yoga produces nadi shuddhi (purification of all channels of communication) and mala shuddhi (eradication of factors that disturb balanced working of body and mind).

According to Swami Kuvalayananda, Yoga helps cultivation of positive health through three integral steps:

1. Cultivation of correct psychological attitudes (maitri, karuna, mudita and upekshanam towards those who are sukha, duhkha, punya and apunya),

2. Reconditioning of neuro-muscular and neuro-glandular system – in fact, the whole body – enabling it to withstand stress and strain better,

3. Laying great emphasis on appropriate diet conducive to such a peak state of health, and encouraging the natural processes of elimination through various processes of nadi shuddhi or mala shuddhi.

To live a healthy life it is important to do healthy things and follow a healthy lifestyle. The modern world is facing a pandemic of lifestyle disorders that require changes to be made consciously by individuals themselves. Yoga places great importance on a proper and healthy lifestyle whose main components are:

1. Achar –Yoga stresses the importance of healthy activities such as exercise and recommends asana, pranayama and kriya on a regular basis. Cardio-respiratory health is one of the main by-products of such healthy activities.

2. Vichar –Right thoughts and right attitude towards life is vital for well being. A balanced state of mind is obtained by following the moral restraints and ethical observances (yama-niyama). As Mahatma Gandhi said, "there is enough in this world for everyone's need but not enough for any one person's greed".

3. Ahar – Yoga emphasises need for a healthy, nourishing diet that has an adequate intake of fresh water along with a well balanced intake of fresh food, green salads, sprouts, unrefined cereals and fresh fruits. It is important to be aware of the need for a satwica diet, prepared and served with love and affection.

4. Vihar – Proper recreational activities to relax body and mind are essential for good health. This includes proper relaxation, maintaining quietude of action-speech-thoughts and group activities wherein one loses the sense of individuality. Karma Yoga is an excellent method for losing the sense of individuality and gaining a sense of universality.

According to Yogacharini Meenakshi Devi Bhavanani, Director ICYER at Ananda Ashram in Pondicherry, Yoga has a step-by-step method for producing and maintaining perfect health at all levels of existence. She explains that social behaviour is first optimized through an understanding and control of the lower animal nature (pancha yama) and development and enhancement of the higher humane nature (pancha niyama). The body is then strengthened, disciplined, purified, sensitized, lightened, energized and made obedient to the higher will through asana. Universal pranic energy that flows through body-mind-emotions- spirit continuum is intensified and controlled through pranayama using breath control as a method to attain controlled expansion of the vital cosmic energy. The externally oriented senses are explored, refined, sharpened and made acute, until finally the individual can detach themselves from sensory impressions at will through pratyahara. The restless mind is then purified, cleansed, focused and strengthened through concentration (dharana). If these six steps are thoroughly understood and practiced then the seventh, dhyana or meditation (a state of union of the mind with the object of contemplation) is possible. Intense meditation produces samadhi, or the enstatic feeling of Union, Oneness with the Universe. This is the perfect state of integration or harmonious health.

MODERN MEDICINE AND YOGA:

Though modern medicine may not share all of these concepts with Yoga, it is to be seen that there are a great many 'meeting points' for the construction of a healthy bridge between them. Both modern medicine and Yoga understand the need for total health and even the Word Health Organization has recently added a new dimension to the modern understanding of health by including spiritual health in its definition of the "state of health'. Spiritual health is an important element of Yoga and now that even the WHO has come around to understanding this point of view, there is hope for a true unification of these two systems. Modern medicine has the ultimate aim and goal of producing a state of optimum physical and mental health thus ultimately leadings to the optimum well being of the individual. Yoga also aims at the attainment of mental and physical well being though the methodology does differ. While modern medicine has a lot to offer humankind in its treatment and management of acute illness, accidents and communicable diseases, Yoga has a lot to offer in terms of preventive, promotive and rehabilitative methods in addition to many management methods to tackle modern illnesses. While modern science looks outward for the cause of all ills, the Yogi searches the depth of his own self. This two way search can lead us to many answers for the troubles that plague modern man. The Shiva-Samhita lists the characters of a fully qualified disciple (shishya) as follows. "Endowed with great energy and enthusiasm, intelligent, heroic, learned in the scriptures, free from delusion..." Doesn't a true modern medical scientist require these very same qualities?

YOGA AND SOCIAL LIFE:

The science and art of Yoga, has for millennia guided man in his search for truth. Even in his personal and social life, Yoga has given him the tools and techniques with which he can find happiness, spiritual realization and social harmony. Various Yogic concepts have guided man towards shaping his life and the interpersonal relationships in his social life. The Yogic concepts of samatvam (mental and emotional equanimity) and stitha prajna (the even minded, balanced human being) give us role models that we may strive to emulate.

An understanding of the pancha klesha (five psycho-physiological afflictions) and their role in the creation of stress and the stress response help us to know ourselves better and understand the how's and why's of what we do. The concept of the pancha kosha (the five layered existence of man as elucidated in the Taittiriya Upanishad) helps us to understand that we have more than only the physical existence and also gives us an insight into the role of the mind in causation of our physical problems as well as psychosomatic disorders. All of these concepts help us to look at life with a different perspective (yoga drishti) and strive to evolve consciously towards becoming Humane Beings. The concept of vairagya (dispassion or detachment) when understood and cultivated enables us to be dispassionate to the dwandwa (the pairs of opposites) such as praise-blame, hot-cold and the pleasant-unpleasant situations; that are part and parcel of our existence in this life.

The regular practice of Yoga as a 'Way of Life' (as defined by Yogamaharishi Dr Swami Gitananda Giri Guru Maharaj) helps us reduce the levels of physical, mental and emotional stress. This Yogic 'way of life' lays emphasis on right thought, right action, right reaction and right attitude. In short Pujya Swamiji defined Yogic living as "right-use-ness of body, emotions and mind".

The pancha yama and pancha niyama provide a strong moral and ethical foundation for our personal and social life. They guide our attitudes with regard to the right and wrong in our life and in relation to our self, our family unit and the entire social system. The yama-niyama provide a strong moral and ethical foundation for our personal and social life. They guide our attitudes with regard to the right and wrong in our life and in relation to our self, our family unit and the entire social system. These changes in our attitude and behaviour will go a long way in helping to prevent the very causes of stress in our life.

The pancha yama consisting of ahimsa (non – violence), satya (truthfulness), asteya (non-stealing), brahmacharya (proper channeling of creative impulse) and aparigraha (non – coveted-ness) are the "do not's" in a Yoga Sadhaka's life. Do not kill, do not be untruthful, do not steal, do not waste your god given creativity and do not covet that which does not belong to you. These guide us to say a big "NO" to our lower self and the lower impulses of violence etc. When we apply these to our life we can definitely have better personal and social relationships as social beings.

The pancha niyama consisting of saucha (cleanliness), santhosha (contentment), tapa (leading a disciplined life of austerity), svadhyaya (introspectional self analysis), and ishwara pranidhana (developing a sense of gratitude to the divine self) guide us with "DO'S" - do be clean, do be contented, do be disciplined, do self - study (introspection) and do be thankful to the divine for all of his blessings. They help us to say a big "YES" to our higher self and the higher impulses. Definitely a person with such qualities is a God-send to humanity. Even when we are unable to live the yama-niyama completely, even the attempt by us to do so will bear fruit and make each one of us a better person and help us to be of value to those around us and a valuable person to live with in our family and society. These are values which need to be introduced to the youth in order to make them aware and conscious of these wonderful concepts of daily living which are qualities to be imbibed with joy and not learnt with fear or compulsion.

Living a happy and healthy life on all planes is possible through the unified practice of Hatha Yoga especially when performed consciously and with awareness. Asana help to develop strength, flexibility, will power, good health, and stability and thus when practiced as a whole give a person a 'stable and unified strong personality'. Pranayama helps us to control our emotions which are linked to breathing and the pranamaya kosha (the vital energy sheath or body). Slow, deep and rhythmic breathing helps to control stress and overcome emotional hang-ups. The inner aspects of Yoga such as dharana and dhyana help us to focus our mid and dwell in it and thus help us to channel our creative energy in a wholistic manner towards the right type of evolutionary activities. They help us to understand ourselves better and in the process become better humans in this social world.

The adoption of Bhakti Yoga enables us to realise the greatness of the Divine and understand our puniness as compared to the power of the Divine or nature. We realize that we are but 'puppets on a string' following his commands on the stage of the world and then perform our activities with the intention of them being an offering to the divine and gratefully receive HIS/HER/ITS blessings.

DEVELOPING ESSENTIAL QUALITIES OF A GOOD HUMAN BEING

The universe is the Divine, nature is the Divine and every being is the Divine. You are the Divine and the Divine is you. Of course we must be careful that we don't go on an ego trip by misunderstanding this reality. The Divine is 'that' which is beyond name and form yet manifests to us through every name and form dear to us. He, She, It manifests to me personally through my father, my mother, my wife, my children, my students, my patients, my teachers, anyone and anything I choose to hold dear to my heart. Yoga is the dearest thing I hold to my heart and so for me the Divine is Yoga and Yoga is the Divine.

Patanjali says that the Divine, or iswara, is beyond the impurities of klesha (affliction or poison) and fructifications of the karma. He also implies in the Yoga Darshan that 'we' can become 'that' divinity itself when we rid ourselves of the impurities that prevent that awareness. Every yoganga, every part of Yoga, every part of life itself is a state of being, a state wherein we are a pure vehicle for the universal nature to manifest in its totality. The Divine is therefore for me a 'state of being'. If you are in that state, everything is Divine. On the other hand if we are not in such a state, then everything seems to be non-Divine.

Some of the important human qualities one must try and develop in the Yogic life are:

• Always be a good learner, ready to learn every moment

• Develop a strong self-introspective ability

• Be disciplined and dedicated towards the cause of Yoga

• Try to develop an understanding of the holistic nature of Yoga physiology, philosophy and psychology along with a strong desire for spiritual evolution

• Be willing to learn from all situations

- Learn not to have an, "I know it all!" attitude.

- Develop a sense of empathy for others

- Be willing to sublimate our own EGO

- Have a good sense of humour and laugh at yourself without reservation

- Try to motivate others by self-example and lead the way as a true acharya.

- Always have devotion to the guru who has guided you for guru droha or treachery to one's guru is considered the worst sin.

- Do your best and leave the rest for everything happens only for our spiritual evolution.

CONCLUSION:

Love for Yoga is the key component of a Yoga life. Of course, joy and fun are part of the Yoga life at all times. Develop an ardent desire to evolve on the path towards oneness and keep working on it non stop. Compassion, empathy and love are important dynamics that are to be worked on while petty egocentric stuff needs to be kept at the bottom of the pile. The ability to sublimate one's individuality for the sake of the group is an important part of the Yoga life. Constant growth through satsangha is very useful, and being open to correction and change at all times is a must. We need to remember that the guru is not just the physical manifestation but is a spirit of guidance that can manifest through so many vehicles. One must be constant on the lookout for its manifestation as such a spirit may manifest through our partner, our children, our neighbours, our students, our friends and often through our worst enemies too. I have found that people who consider me their worst enemy have actually helped my growth more than some who have always been caring and considerate. The ones who always looking for chances to degrade me keep me on my toes, and make me do the best I can without fail. They are the stimulant that enables the best to flower through me. When they play such a great role in my life, is it not right that I thank them for being a manifestation of the guru spirit too?

Yoga is not just performing some contortionist poses or huffing and puffing some pranayama or sleeping our way through any so-called meditation. It is an integrated way of life in which awareness and consciousness play a great part in guiding our spiritual evolution through life in the social system itself and not in some remote cave in the mountains or hut in the forest. As my beloved Guru-Father Pujya Swamiji Gitananda Giri Guru Maharaj said "Yoga is the science and art of right- useness of body, emotions and mind".

Through the dedicated practice of Yoga as a way of life, we can become a truly balanced humane being (sthita prajna) with the following qualities as described in the Bhagavad Gita:

• Beyond passion, fear and anger. (II.56)

• Devoid of possessiveness and egoism. (II.71)

• Firm in understanding and un-bewildered. (V.20)

• Engaged in doing good to all beings. (V.25)

• Friendly and compassionate to all. (XII.13)

• Having no expectation, pure and skilful in action. (XII.16)

The Yogi wishes peace and happiness not only for himself, but also for all beings on all the different planes of existence. He is not an "individualist" seeking salvation for only himself but on the contrary is an "universalist" seeking to live life in the proper evolutionary manner to the best of his ability and with care and concern for his human brethren as well as all beings on all planes of existence.

"Om, loka samasta sukhino bhavanthu sarve janaha sukhino bhavanthu" "Om shanti, shanti, shanti Om"

RECOMMENDED READING:

1. A Primer of Yoga Theory. Dr Ananda Balayogi Bhavanani. Dhivyananda Creations, Iyyanar Nagar, Pondicherry. 2008.

2. A Yogic Approach to Stress. Dr Ananda Balayogi Bhavanani.. Dhivyananda Creations, Iyyanar Nagar, Pondicherry. (2nd edition) 2008.

3. Ancient Yoga and Modern Science. TR Anantharaman. Mushiram Manoharlal Publishers Pvt Ltd, New Delhi. 1996

4. Ashtanga Yoga of Patanjali. Dr Swami Gitananda Giri. Edited by Meenakshi Devi Bhavanani. Satya Press, Pondicherry.1995

5. Back issues of International Journal of Yoga Therapy. Journal of the International Association of Yoga Therapists, USA. www.iayt.org

6. Back issues of Yoga Life, Monthly Journal of ICYER at Ananda Ashram, Pondicherry. www.icyer.com

7. Back issues of Yoga Mimamsa. Journal of Kaivalyadhama, Lonavla, Maharashtra.

8. Four Chapters on Freedom. Commentary on Yoga Sutras of Patanjali by Swami Satyananda Saraswathi, Bihar School of Yoga, Munger, India. 1999

9. Frankly speaking. Dr Swami Gitananda Giri. Edited by Meenakshi Devi Bhavanani. Satya Press, Pondicherry.1995

10. Mudras. Dr Swami Gitananda Giri. Revised by Ananda Balayogi Bhavanani. Satya Press, Pondicherry.2006

11. Pranayama: The Fourth limb of Ashtanga Yoga. Dr Swami Gitananda Giri, Meenakshi Devi Bhavanani, Ananda Balayogi Bhavanani and Devasena Bhavanani. Satya Press, Pondicherry.2008

12. Srimad Bhagavad Gita by Swami Swarupananda. Advaita Ashrama, Kolkata. 2007

13. The Forceful Yoga (being the translation of the Hathayoga Pradipika, Gheranda Samhita and Siva Samhita). Translated into English by Pancham Sinh, Rai Bahadur Srisa Chandra Vasu and Romanized and edited by Dr GP Bhatt. Mothilal Banarsidas Publishers Private Limited, Delhi. 2004.

14.The Supreme Yoga: Yoga Vashista. Swami Venkatesananda. Mothilal Banarsidas Publishers Pvt Ltd. Delhi.2007

15. www.icyer.com

16. www.rishiculture.in

Bhavanani AB. Yoga: The ideal way of life. Yoga Mimamsa 2013; 44(4): 314-25.

17. Yoga and Sports. Swami Gitananda Giri and Meenakshi Devi Bhavanani. Satya Press, Pondicherry.1991

18. Yoga for Health and Healing. Dr Ananda Balayogi Bhavanani. Dhivyananda Creations, Iyyanar Nagar, Pondicherry. 2007

19. Yoga Therapy Notes. Dr Ananda Balayogi Bhavanani. Dhivyananda Creations, Iyyanar Nagar, Pondicherry. 2007

20. Yoga: Step by Step. Dr Swami Gitananda Giri. Satya Press, Pondicherry.1975

Yogachariya Jnandev Giri
Founder and Senior Sanatan & Gitananda Yoga Teacher

D. Pharmacy, B.SC., M.SC. Preksha Meditation & Yoga, 3000hrs Intensive
YTT at ICYER, India, MS Psychotherapy & Counselling

Surender Saini now known as Yogachariya Jnandev was born in a typical Hindu family. He grew up under the guidance and blessings of his virtuous parents, loving and caring two brothers and a sister. This gave Jnandev a strong foundation for a yogic ethical and moral lifestyle. He also had a great influence on his late Nana (grandfather), who was a great bhajan singer and spiritual storyteller. He will also get Jnandev to read Ramayana, Mahabharata and other Hindu epic stories. This planted some seeds of spirituality, Hinduism and yoga in Jnandev's young mind.

Jnandev began his career as a Pharmacist, but he did not enjoy that for too long. He found it not much of help in helping people to be healthy or happy. So, he went back to further education. Jnandev had a great interest in science and hence went on to his graduation in Maths, Physics and Chemistry. These aspects of studies have given Jnandev a much greater understanding of many yogic ideas and principles from scientific perspectives.

In 1995 during the Pharmacy course, he met a friend who gave him initiation into some concentration practices, relaxation techniques and a few asanas or postures to learn hypnosis. After a few months of Trataka, relaxation practices and some visualisation, Jnandev felt drawn to learn more and more about hatha yoga, meditation and relaxation techniques and followed various ashrams, yoga centres, yoga shalas as and when he could. Since then, he tries to do some of his sadhana every day.

At the end of his graduation, he decided to follow the path of civil services in India and was preparing for competition exams for it. During this period his Sadhana also got deeper and deeper and he felt drawn to finding the true meaning of life through yoga. In this quest, he arrived at Jain Vishwa Bharati University, Ladnun and 2000 and completed his MSC in Preksha Meditation and Yoga as a gold medallist. Here he was blessed by the presence of his Guru Sthita Prajna Ji, who guided Jnandev on every level of his sadhana.

Also, Jnandev spend most of his time in one of the richest libraries, where he managed to read or study many original scriptures and manuscripts.

This was the time were Jnandev also started to write. Since 2000, Jnandev had written many articles, and research papers in India. This was the beginning point of this yoga course. Since then, Jnandev has visited and lived in many ashrams, and yoga institutes to learn, practice and grow in his sadhana.

From 2003 to 2006 Jnandev worked in one of the most reputed schools in Jaipur (M.G.P.S, Vidyadhar Nagar, Jaipur). This gave Jnandev a new opportunity to explore various aspects of Hatha Yoga practices to benefit young children. Jnandev learned, followed and taught various hatha yoga kriya sets and asanas and mudras from beginners to advance levels during this time.

During this time to understand our mind from a modern perspective, Jnandev also completed Masters in Psychotherapy and Counselling course (distance learning).

2006-07 Jnandev in search of advancing his sadhana and yogic development arrived at Ananda Ashram, Puducherry. The six-month advanced yoga teacher training course under the guidance of his now Guru Ammaji Meenakshi Devi and Dr Ananda Balayogi Bhavanani completed Jnandev's journey of search for true authentic yoga. This intensive six-month course in Gitananda Rishiculture Ashtanga Yoga gave a new life or birth to present Jnandev. Ammaji also gave the name and title

'Yogachariya Jnandev' to Surender at the end of the course, which he uses in most parts of his life now.

All this time, Jnandev managed to not only do his Sadhana regularly but kept writing his notes, practices, understanding and experiences of various practices, philosophical ideas and principles.

After meeting with Yogacharini Deepika, Jnandev arrived in the UK in 2008. In 2009 he established Yoga Satsanga Ashram, Wales, UK and in 2010-11 started to run the first foundation course in Yoga compiled from all these writings and teachings Jnandev was working on since 2000. Since then, Jnandev has authored 9 books and more to be published along with compiling Yoga Teacher Training Course, Kids Yoga Teacher Training Course, Yoga Therapy Course and many other such courses with the full assistance of Yogacharini Deepika.

The Sanatan Yoga primarily follows Gitananda Yoga but also has a great in-put of teachings and blessings of Jain Vishwas Bharati, Hatha Yoga Guru Balendu Giriji, Mahavira Nathaji and many more divine souls. Blessings of Ammaji and Dr Ananda has kept, Jnandev on this straight path of Yoga.

Yogachariya Jnandev met Yogacharini Deepika at Ananda ashram. They both had three lovely boys, growing up in the Ashram and helping to grow and evolve every day. Since Jnandev came to UK Deepika has been a great guide and contributor to his yoga journey. Deepika has worked very sincerely in helping Jnandev to bring this course to present form.

Since 2021 Yogachariya Jnandev has founded Gurukula – Home of Sanatan Yoga Sadhana and Education, Portugal.

May Divine and GURU (one who shows us the path to self-realisation and guides us from darkness to light) always bless us all together on this path of yoga to grow spiritually.

May the Divine and Guru give us strength and courage to follow this path of discipline which can lead us to the union of body-mind-soul.

May the divine bless all with SAT-CHIT-ANANDA (divine love and bliss).

Yogacharya Dr. ANANDA BALAYOGI BHAVANANI
MBBS, ADY, DPC, DSM, PGDFH, PGDY, FIAY, MD (Alt.Med), C-IAYT, DSc (Yoga)

Yogacharya Dr. Ananda Balayogi Bhavanani is Director of the Centre for Yoga Therapy Education and Research (CYTER), and Professor of Yoga Therapy at the Sri Balaji Vidyapeeth, Pondicherry (www.sbvu.ac.in).

He is also Chairman of the International Centre for Yoga Education and Research at Ananda Ashram, Pondicherry, India (www.icyer.com) and Yoganjali Natyalayam, the premier institute of Yoga and Carnatic Music and Bharatanatyam in Pondicherry (www.rishiculture.in). He is son and successor of the internationally acclaimed Yoga team of Yogamaharishi Dr. Swami Gitananda Giri Guru Maharaj and Yogacharini Kalaimamani Ammaji, Smt Meenakshi Devi Bhavanani.

A recipient of the prestigious DSc (Yoga) from SVYASA Yoga University in January 2019, he is a Gold Medallist in Medical Studies (MBBS) with postgraduate diplomas in both Family Health (PGDFH) as well as Yoga (PGDY) and the Advanced Diploma in Yoga under his illustrious parents in 1991-93. A

Fellow of the Indian Academy of Yoga, he has authored 19 DVDs and 26 books on Yoga as well as published nearly 300 papers, compilations and abstracts on Yoga and Yoga research in National and International Journals. His literary works have more than 2800 Citations, with an h-Index of 26 and an i10-Index of 56. In addition, he is a Classical Indian Vocalist, Percussionist, Music Composer and Choreographer of Indian Classical Dance.

In recent years he has travelled abroad 20 times and conducted invited talks, public events, workshops and retreats and been major presenter at Yoga conferences in the UK, USA, Italy, Czech Republic, South Africa, Germany, Switzerland, Malaysia, Canada, Australia and New Zealand.

He is an Honorary Advisor to International Association of Yoga Therapists (www.iayt.org), Australasian Association of Yoga Therapists (www.yogatherapy.org.au), World Yoga Foundation (www.worldyogafoundation.in) and Gitananda Yoga Associations worldwide (www.rishiculture.in).

A recognized PhD guide for Yoga Therapy he was recognized as an IAYT Certified Yoga Therapist (C-IAYT) by the International Association of Yoga Therapists, USA in 2016. It is notable that he is the first Indian to receive this honour.

He is member of numerous expert committees of the Ministry of AYUSH including its Steering Committee of the Yoga Certification Board, National Board for Promotion of Yoga and Naturopathy, Scientific Advisory Committee & Standing Finance Committees of CCRYN, Expert Committees for Celebration of International Yoga Day and the National Yoga & Diabetes program. He is Consultant Resource Person for the WHO and its Collaborative Centre in Traditional Medicine (Yoga) at MDNIY, New Delhi. He is also Joint Secretary of the Indian Yoga Association (www.yogaiya.in) and Senior Vice President of National Yogasana Sports Federation (https://yogasanasport.in).

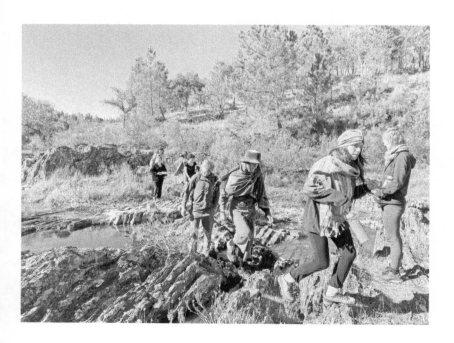

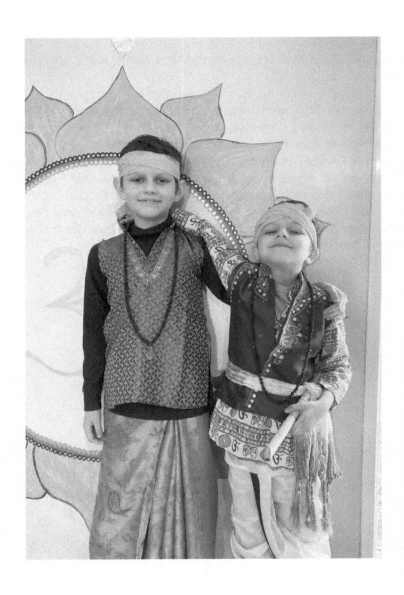

Yoga Moral Stories

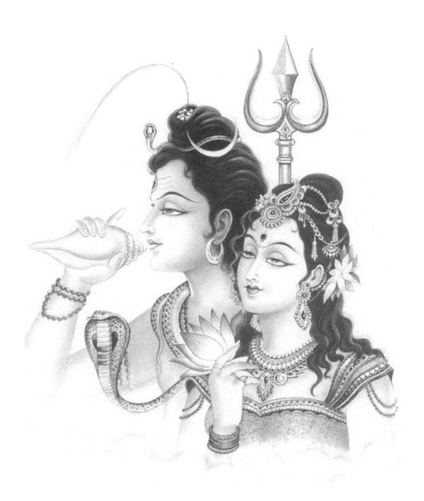

Our World- Manifestation of Our Own Mind

Once a young man riding a horse arrived at entrance gate of a village in India.

There was an old watch man sitting at near the gate.

Young man said, I am thinking to live in this village. Can you tell me about nature of the people in this village? Are they peaceful and kind people or not?

Old man asked him, first you tell me about the people of the village you left before you came here.

Young man said, don't even remind me about those people, they make me angry. They were terribly bad people. They had no peace or love.

Old man said that, I have 70 years of experience with the people of this village. They are worst then the people of last village. You must go and find a better village to live.

After a while another family arrived at the entrance of village. They asked the old man, same question. They wanted to live in that village and wanted to know about the people in the village.

Old man asked them the same question too

The family said, the village we left had most amazing, kind and loving people. Our eyes are still full of tears and we feel sad to leave them.

Old man said, you will find this village even more loving, kind and peaceful. Come and live with us. I have 70 years of experience living with the people of this village.

Moral- Peace, love and goodness is within us. If we are kind, loving and caring, then people around us are also kind, loving and caring. Our world is simply manifestation of who we are within ourselves.

A thief and Fakira

A fakira was living in a little hut in Japan. Once around mid night, someone broke through his door and entered the Hut.

Fakir asked in the dark, who is there? What can I do for you?

Thief was a little frightened and got a knife out.

Fakir said, you don't need a knife, no one bad living here.

Thief was even more scared now, and said, I am a thief, I am here to steal your money.

Fakir said, How sad it is to see, you have to come out at this time. How terrible your life situation must be to make you do this.

Come and take the money, I have very little said the Fakir.

Thief took the money and was about to leave. Fakir said can you leave few coins behind please, so I can get few things in morning.

Thief left few coins and about to walk out of the door.

Fakir asked him again, you have taken the money, at least you should say thank you.

Frightened thief said thank you and walked away in dark.

After several months thief was caught red handed during a theft. Many people came forward to witness about many stealings he has committed.

The Judge also came to know about the stealing incident at Fakir's hut.

Fakir was asked to verify if he has stolen anything from his place. Fakir was very respected and well known. Everyone knew that his witness will be very much valued. Thief was very frightened as he knew that Fakir has witnessed him stealing in his place.

Judge asked the Fakir, do you know this man?

Fakir, said yes. He is one my friends. He came to visit me few months ago, and took some money. He said thank you in return before leaving.

Thief was surprised and came to see the Fakir after completing his punishment and asked for forgiveness.

Moral- Our experiences and perceptions are depending on who we are within ourselves. If we are in deep peace and equanimity within, there is nothing bad or wrong out there. Seek for peace, love and joy within your heart and go deep within to remove all that is bad or immoral.

Jagadguru Shankaracharya and Sananda

This is a beautiful story about Jagadguru Shankaracharya, and his disciple Sananda. He was uneducated and hence was unable to understand the teachings of his Guru. But whenever Shankarachariya delivered the Satsanga, he would listen sincerely with wholeheartedly attention and faith.

One day Sanada was busy washing his Guru's clothes by the other side of river. It was the time for him to deliver his teachings. His disciplines requested, "Guruji please begin the satsanga as it is time to begin."

Shankaracharya replied, "Let us wait; Sananda is not here."

His disciples urged, "But Guruji, he cannot understand anything,"

Shakaracharya said, "That is true; still, he listens with great faith and so I do not wish to disappoint him."

To reveal the power of faith, Shankaracharya called, "walk straight to me now Sanada".

Hearing his Guru's wish, without hesitation we walked straight across the river on the water and arrived at his Guru. As we walked across the river, lotus flowers blossomed under his feet to support his Guru Bhakti. Sanada offered his greetings and blessings to his Guru's feet. At that time he chanted the Guru-Shrotram (verses in praise of guru) in Sanskrita in a most sophisticated manner.

That day he was named "Padmapada" due to the lotus flowers supporting him crossing the river.

Moral:- Even if we listen the adhyatmic teachings and the satsanga (sacred dialogues about truth) we gradually develop shraddha, purity, and attain Jnana Yoga.

No Dharma is Lower or Higher

This story illustrates that no duty is pure or impure and lower or higher. It is the consciousness and intention behind the Karma that determines its quality and worth. This story was told to Yudhishthara by Sage Markendeya in the Vana Parva of the Mahabharat.

Once upon a time a young sanyasi went into the forest, where he meditated and performed tapas for a many years.

One day a crow's droppings fell upon him from the tree above whilst he was in meditation. It disturbed his meditation and he looked angrily at the bird. The bird fell dead on the ground from the curse of his anger.

The sanyasi realized that he had gained mystical powers as a result of his tapas. He was filled with pride.

Later, he went to a house to beg for alms. The housewife came to the door, and requested him to wait a while, since she was looking after her diseased husband.

This angered the Sannyasi and he looked at her with anger, thinking, "You worthless woman, how dare you make a sannyasi wait! You do not know my powers."

The woman replied, "You do not need to look at me with such anger. I am not a crow to be burnt by your glance."

The sannyasi was shocked, and asked how she knew about what he was thinking?

The woman said she did not practice any tapas like him, but has performed all her duties with devotion and dedication. By virtue of it, she had been blessed with the inner-light and was able to read his mind.

She then suggested that he should meet a righteous butcher who lived in the town of Mithila, and said that he would answer his questions on dharma.

The sanyasi overcame his initial hesitation of speaking to a low caste butcher and came to see him in Mithila.

The righteous butcher then explained to him that we all have our respective swa-dharma, based upon our past karmas and experience. But if we fulfil our natural dharma, and also renounce the desire for personal gain and rise above the fleeting happiness and misery arising from the outcomes of our actions. By doing so, we will purify ourselves and advance to the next class of dharma.

By fulfilling our dharma or performing our duties and not running away from them, the mind gradually evolves from its present gross worldly consciousness to eternal divine consciousness.

Gods and Demons (a story from Kenopanishad)

Once upon a time, there was a prolonged war between the devatas (heavenly gods) and the daityas (demons from the nether region). Eventually, the devatas won the battle with the grace Supreme Divine. All the Gods out of pride thought that they won the battle because of their own strength. Parmatman manifested in heavenly plane in form an effulgent Yaksha to teach the lesson to the gods.

When Indra saw the Yaksha, he felt insecure and intimidated. He sent Agni-Deva (the fire god) to find out who this Yaksha was. The Agni-deva challenged the yaksha by saying that he is the god of fire and can burn the entire world in minutes. Yaksha placed a little grass straw in the middle, and asked if Agni-deva could burn it. Agni-Deva laughed and tried to burn the grass with his mighty fires. Agni-deva gradually felt cold and defeated and he ran back to Indra.

Next Indra sent Vayu Deva (the wind god) to enquire who this Yaksha was. Vayu Deva said out of pride, "I am Vayu Deva and possess the power to blow everything away and turn it all upside down in minutes." Yaksha put a little piece of grass and asked the Vayu Deva to blow it away or turn over if he can. Vayu full of pride, tried his best, but couldn't move it even a little. Defeated, and exhausted he also returned back to Indra.

Indra was raged and came to challenge the Yaksha himself. But the Yaksha disappeared and in his place Goddess Uma, the Yogamaya power of Supreme Divine was seating in his place. Indra asked, "O divine Mother Goddess, please tell me who that powerful Yaksha was?" She replied, "O thoughtless and ignorant child, how couldn't you recognise Him? Your pride had blinded your farsightedness. He was your Supreme Father, the creator, the source of energy and light, without him you are all powerless." Realising this Indra begged for forgiveness.

A Frog and the Ocean

This is a story from Hindu Philosphical phrase, 'kupa-manduka-nyaya – the logic of frog'. There was a frog living in a deep well, unaware of the world outside the walls of the well. Once a frog from the ocean got washed off and fell into the well.

Frog from the well asked, "How big is the ocean, where you lived?" Frog from the ocean replied, "it is huge and has no beginning or no end." The frog from the well said, "Is it five times bigger than this well?" The frog from the ocean said, no it is much bigger. So the frog from the well said it 10 times larger? Frog from the ocean said, no it is much larger. Curious frog from the well said, "Is it 100 times bigger than?. The frog from the ocean said, no 100 times is nothing in compared to the ocean. It is much more larger. The frog from the well said, "I know all this time you are lying, as nothing can be larger than this well as he lived all his life within the boundaries of the well."

The frog from the well couldn't comprehend anything larger than the well in which he was living.

This teaching is well explained by Noble laureate and French physiologist, Alexis Carrel, in his book, Man the Unknown. He states: "Our mind has a natural tendency to reject the things that do not fit into the frame of scientific or philosophical beliefs of our time. After all, scientists are only human. They are saturated with the prejudices of their environment and epoch. They willingly believe that facts which cannot be explained by current theories do not exist. At present times, scientists still look upon telepathy and other metaphysical phenomena as illusions. Evident facts having an unorthodox appearance are suppressed."

Story of Tulsidasa

A young man, Tulsidas was madly in love with his wife. Once she went to visit her parents for few days. They lived in a village across a river stream. It was very bad weather with heavy rain and storm, but Tulsidas was feeling restless and eager to see his wife.

He decided to go and see her right away that night. It was dark and the boatman was not willing to take him across the river. Tulsidas saw something floating nearby and without even thinking twice, he clung to it and crossed the river.

When he reached her parents' house, it was late and felt hesitant to wake everyone up. His wife lived in the room on the second floor in her parents' house. He saw a rope hanging from the window, he climbed up to get to her room with the help the rope.

She was surprised to see him there and asked him how he had managed to come to see her that late in such terrible weather. He detailed all as it happened. When they looked at the window, there was no rope, but a snake which Tulsidas assumed to be a rope. Also what Tulsidas assumed to be a floating log was a dead body. His desire to see his wife was so strong that he was totally blinded to see the reality.

His wife was furious and said to him, "You desire to see me, a body made of flesh and blood so intensely that you lost your sight. If you could have such an intense desire to see the Divine, you will attain Him and be free of the cycle of birth and death."

Her words changed his life and Tulidas left home and renounced a household life. He totally detached himself from the worldly desires and pleasures and engaged himself in devotion to Lord Rama. Later he become one of the great saint and poet and wrote Ramayama.

He wrote in Ramayana, "As a lustful man desires a beautiful woman, and as a greedy person desires wealth, may my mind and senses constantly desire Lord Rama."

A Guru and Shishya on How to Liberate from the Maya

Once in the forests of Himalayas, lived a Guru and Shishya in their ashram. The guru was wise and known of true knowledge on the path, and practices to attain liberation.

One day the curious disciple asked his guru, "please master tell me how to attain freedom the worldly attachments, and illusion (Maya)."

The master said, "I will tell you the truth when it is the right time."

The student was disappointed for a moment, but knew that his master knows the truth about liberation from prison of maya and hence waited patiently.

One day the student went into the forest to pick some dry wood for the Havan (fire ceremony). Suddenly he heard his master shouting out loud for help. He heard his Guru's voice in pain and begging for help.

The student ran as fast as he could, following his guru's voice. He had all sorts of thoughts like "is my guru being attacked by a tiger or are there robbers in ashram attacking my guru?"

Soon he arrived at the ashram, sweating and heart pounding. He saw his Guru caught in a tree. He was surprised to find that his guru was hugging the tree and asking for help to be freed from the tree.

The Student said, "Master, it seems you are holding on to the tree and nothing is stopping you to be free other than your own grip and misunderstanding or avidya. Please ease your hands and let yourself be free of the tree."

Guru smiled and said, "True my dear student, you are also holding on to your misconceptions that you are caught in the maya of world. Situations, material objects, thoughts, feelings, karma and their fruits, as well as the subtlest samaskaras are not holding on to you. You are holding on them. Let go and know that the Atman and Parmatman are only True Reality that exist eternally. Everything else is Maya."

The student realised the truth and offered his gratitude with true love and bliss.

Does God Exist?

This is a beautiful story of a King and Sadhu regarding perception and existence of the God.

A king once confronted a Sadhu with the statement, "I do not believe in God because I cannot see Him."

The sadhu asked the King to bring a cow. The king happily ordered his servants to bring a cow.

The sadhu then requested the King for the cow to be milked. The king again instructed his servants to do as the sadhu wanted.

The sadhu asked, "O King! Do you believe that this milk, freshly taken out from the cow, contains butter?"

The king said he knows as well as he believes that there is butter in the milk.

The sadhu said, "You cannot see the butter in the milk. Then why do you believe it is there?"

The king replied, "We cannot see it at present because the butter is pervading the milk, but there is a process for seeing it. We need to convert the milk into the yogurt and then churn the yogurt to get the butter out. Then the cutter will be visible."

The sadhu said, "Like the butter in the milk, God is everywhere. If we cannot immediately perceive Him, we should not jump to the conclusion that there is no God. There is a sadhana process for perceiving Him; if we are willing to have faith and follow the process, we will then get a direct perception of God and become God-realized."

Vidurs Love and Devotion for Krishna

Whenever God descends upon the earth, He exhibits His impartial love in His divine Leelas or Amusements.

Before the Mahabharat war, Shree Krishna went to Hastinapur as a Peace messenger to avoid the battle and to explore the possibility of forming an agreement between the Kauravas and Pandavas.

The evil Duryodhan proudly prepared offered Him a meal with fifty-six different items (chappan-bhoga). Shree Krishna rejected his hospitality and instead went to the humble hut of Vidura and his wife.

They both had been yearning deeply for the opportunity to serve their beloved Lord. Vidurani was overjoyed on receiving the Supreme Lord at her home. All she had to offer Krishna was bananas. Her intellect so absorbed in loving sentiments and pealed a banana and dropped the banana and offered banana peels to Krishna.

Krishna also absorbed in Bhakti-Bhava started to eat the banana peel blissfully and praised how delicious it was.

The Story of Dadhichi's Sacrifice

Indra, the king of heaven was once driven out of his Swarga Loka by a demon called Vritrasura. The demon could not be killed by any weapon known till then because of a Boon.

Indra came to Lord Shiv seeking for help, who took him to Lord Vishnu. Vishnu revealed to Indra that the only weapon that could kill Vritrasura was a thunderbolt made from the bones of the sage Dadhichi.

Indra then begged Sage Dadhichi to make the ultimate sacrifice of laying down his life so that his bones could be used for making the thunderbolt.

Dadhichi accepted the request, but desired to first go on a pilgrimage to all the holy rivers. Indra then brought together all the waters of the holy rivers to Naimisharanya, thereby allowing the sage to have his wish fulfilled without further loss of time.

Dadhichi then gave up his body by the means of yogic practises. The thunderbolt made from his bones was then used to defeat the demon Vritrasura, allowing Indra to regain his place as the king of the Swarga Loka.

Arjuna and Krishna - Bhakti the Path of True Divine Love

Once Arjuna and Krishna were in discussion on various aspects of Bhakti or divine love. Krishna wanted Arjuna to realise the true meaning of Bhakti and hence took him to a little village near Indraprastha.

They both disguised as two young girls and came at a door of little hut. In this hut, a poor old woman known as Pingalai, a great devotee of Krishna lived.

Both the girls requested Pingalai if they can stay with her for a night, as it was getting dark, and they both were also tired after a long journey. Pingalai welcomed them in her hut and offered the food she had.

On one of the walls in the hut, Pingalai has a beautiful picture of Kanha (baby Krishna), who she loves and worships. There were also three swords hanging below the picture of smaller, medium and longer lengths.

Krishna asked her, "dear mother, I see you worship little Krishna, but why do you have three swords of various sizes there too."

Pingalai replied, "I have these three swords to punish three people, who have tortured my darling Kanha."

Arjuna, surprised to hear this, asked who those three people are, who needed be punished for their offences against Krishna.

Krishna further asked, why is that mother?

Pingalai said the smallest of swords is to punish Sudama, as how ignorant he was to feed dry, uncooked rice to my darling Krishna, it would have hurt his lips, tongue and teeth."

Krishna said, "Mother, Sudama was a very poor devotee and friend of Krishna and all he had in his possessions to offer Krishna was three handfuls of rice. He gave his divine, what he had, and so I feel you should forgive him."

Pingalai forgave Sudama as she was asked by Krishna.

Stunned hearing this, Arjuna asked who this second sword is for?

Pingalai further replied, "When Krishna helped Draupadi with providing all the Sarees to protect her from being disrobed, she could have used her own powers to instead. It got stopped when Dushasana fainted of being tired of pulling the sarees off. don't you see that how tiring it was for my darling Kanha to keep sending all those sarees with his beautiful soft hands."

Krishna said, "mother, Draupadi was in such a terrible situation and begged Krishna as her friend and Lord to help her out. Krishna being a Divine, and taken human birth to help people in need, helped Draupadi as his duty and love for his Bhakta."

Pingalai also forgave Draupadi after hearing this out of her love and compassion.

Arjuna was totally shocked and stunned. Krishna further asked, about the third longest sword.

Pingalai replied, "the longest sword is for Arjuna, as he has so many other great masters to be his charioteer and help in the battle. Why he ever needed to get my darling Kanha get involved is such battle."

Krishna said I agree dear mother.

Arjuna was totally shocked to hear that Krishna said I agree mother. Arjuna had many choices. But Krishna become his charioteer out of love and friendship. If you punish Arjuna than Krishna will have friend and Bhakta anymore. Please also forgive Arjuna, suggested Krishna.

Out of love and compassion Pingalai also forgave Arjuna by saying that she will never do anything to hurt her Krishna for any reason and situation.

Arjuna bowed to Krishna and said, "now I understand what true bhakti really means."

Three Robbers and Tri-Gunas

Once a traveller was attacked by three robbers when he was passing through a dense forest.

The first robber said, "let us kill this traveller and rob all his wealth".

The second robber said, "No, let us not kill him. Instead we should tie him to the tree and rob himself all his possessions."

Following the advice of second robber, they tied the traveller and took away all his wealth. After going some distance, the third robber decided to return to free the traveller. He opened the ties of the traveller and show him the path to way out of the forest. He said, "I myself cannot go out of this situation, but you follow this path to get out of th

In this story, first robber was dominated by tamo-guna, the quality of ignorance which was degrading his spirit into sloth, languor, and non-virtue. The second robber was rajo-guna, driven by passion and worldly desires, but has the ability to recognise the value of life. The third robber was of sattva-guna, the quality of goodness, which values the life and endeavour to follow the path of virtue and light in whichever situation or life path it is.

Glossary

Ahamkara ego

Ahimsa Nonviolence, harmlessness (one of the yamas).

Akasha space; ether

Ananda Bliss, joy

Aparigraha Nongreed (one of the yamas).

Arjuna One of the five Pandava back brothers; he whom Lord Krishna Addressed the Bhagavad Gita.

Asanas Yoga postures, 3rd limb of ashtanga yoga.

Ashram Retreat or secluded place, usually where the principles of yoga and meditation are taught and practiced.

Ashtanga Eight limbs

Ashtanga yoga Eightfold path of yoga, Raj Yoga of Patanjali with eight limbs- yamas, Niyamas, etc.

Asmita Ego, individuality, I-am-ness.

Asteya Nonstealing (one of the yamas).

Atma Soul, individual spirit.
Bhakta Devotee.

Bhakti Devotion.

Bhakti yoga The path of devotion.

Brahmacharya Purity, chastity (one of the yamas).

Brahman The absolute. Divinity itself, God as creator.

Buddhi The intellect. Chakras Centers of radiating life force or energy that are located between the base of the spinal column and the crown of the head. Sanskrit for "wheels." There are seven chakras that store and release life force (prana).

Chetana Consciousness, awareness.

Chit Eternal consciousness.

Chit-shakti Mental force governing the subtle dimensions.

Chitta individual consciousness including the subconscious and unconscious levels of mind, memory, thinking, attention, etc.

Chitta-vritti Mental modifications.

Devata Deity

Devi Female deity, goddess.

Dharana From the word dhri meaning "to hold firm," this is concentration or holding the mind to one thought.

Dharma Self-discipline, the life of responsibility and right action.

Dhyana Meditation or contemplation. The process of quieting the mind.

Divya Divine

Doshas Impurities or deformities in body, mind or emotions.

Drashta Seer, observer, awareness.
Drishti Vision.

Gayatri Mantra Vedic mantra of 24 matras or syllables invoking the pure eternal energy.

Gheranda Samhita Traditional yogic text of Rishi Gheranda.

Guru Spiritual teacher.

Hatha yoga It is the yoga of physical well-being, designed to balance body, mind, and spirit.

Indriyas Sense organs.

Ishvar-pranidhana Surrender to God (one of the niyamas).

Iyengar yoga This yoga style focuses on the body and how it works. It is noted for attention to detail, precise alignment of postures, and the use of props.

Jiva Individual life

Jivan Life.

Jnana Knowledge or wisdom.

Jnana yoga The path of knowledge or wisdom.

Kaivalya State of consciousness beyond quality.

Kala Time.

Kama Desires.

Karma Action, law of cause and effect which shapes the destiny of each individual.

Karma yoga The path of action.

Karmendriyas Five physical organs of action- feet, hands, speech, excretory and reproductive organs.
Kirtan Singing holy songs.
Koshas Body, sheaths.
Kriya Motion, movement
Kundalini A cosmic energy in the body that is often compared to a snake lying coiled at the base of the spine, waiting to be awakened. Kundalini is derived from kundala, which means a "ring" or "coil."
Kundalini yoga Chanting and breathing are emphasized over postures in this ancient practice designed to awaken and control the release of kundalini energy.
Laya To dissolve.
Laya yoga Yoga of conscious dissolution of individuality.
Lokas Seven planes of consciousness.
Lord Krishna Because of his great Godly power, Lord Krishna is another of the most commonly worshipped deities in the Hindu faith. He is considered to be the eighth avatar of Lord Vishnu. Shree Krishna delivered Bhagvad Gita on battlefield of Mahabharata to Arjun.
Mala Garland.
Manas Mind.
Mandala A circular geometric design that represents the cosmos and the spirit's pilgrimage. It is a tool in the pilgrimage to enlightenment.
Mantra Sacred chant words.
Mauna Silence.
Maya Illusion.
Mitahara Balanced diet.
Moksha Liberation.
Mudras Hand gestures that direct or control the life current through the body.
Mukti Liberation.
Nada Pranic or psychic sound.
Nadi Channels of pranic/psychic energy flow.

Namaste This Hindu salutation says "the divine in me honors the divine in you." The expression is used on meeting or parting and usually is accompanied by the gesture of holding the palms together in front of the bosom.
Nidra Sleep.
Nirbija Samadhi Final state of smadhi where there is absorption without seed; total dissolution.
Nirvichar Samadhi Transitional state of Samadhi; absorption without reflection.
Nirvikalpa Samadhi Transitional state of Samadhi involving purification of memory, which gives rising to Jnana or true knowledge.
Niyamas In the Yoga Sutras, Patanjali defined five niyamas or observances relating to inner discipline and responsibility. They are purity, contentment, self-discipline, study of the sacred text, and living with the awareness of God.
Om or Aum Mantric word chanted in meditation. Paramahansa Yogananda called it the "vibration of the Cosmic Motor." This one word is interpreted as having three sounds representing creation, preservation, and destruction.
Pancha-klesha Five afflictions – ignorance, ego, attraction, aversion and fear of death.
Patanjali Ancient Rishi who codified the ashtanga yoga known as Yoga-Sutra.
Prakriti Nature.
Prana Life energy, life force, or life current vital energy; inherent vital force pervading every dimension of matter.
Pranava Mantra AUM; primal sound vibration.
Pranava Dhyana Meditation on the mantra AUM.
Pranayama Method of controlling prana or life force through the regulation of breathing.

Pratyahara Withdrawing the senses in order to still the mind as in meditation.

Purusha Individual Soul or spirit.

Raja yoga The path of physical and mental control.

Rishi Realised sage, one who meditate on Self.

Sabeeja Samadhi Absorption with seed where the form of awareness remains.

Sadhaka Spiritual aspirant.

Sadhana Spiritual practice.

Sahaja Spontaneous, easy.

Santosha Contentment (one of the niyamas).

Satya Truthfulness and honesty (one of the yamas).

Samadhi State of absolute bliss, superconsciousness (8th limb of ashtanga yoga).

Shaucha Purity, inner and outer cleanliness (one of the niyamas).

Shat-darshanas Six Ancient Indian philosophies about truth or reality.

Swadhyaya Self-study. The process of inquiring into your own nature, the nature of your beliefs, and the nature of the world's spiritual journey (one of the niyamas).

Swami Title of respect for a spiritual master.

Tamas One of the three gunas; state of inertia or ignorance

Tantra yoga This yoga uses visualization, chanting, asana, and strong breathing practices to awaken highly charged kundalini energy in the body.

Tapas Self-discipline or austerity (one of the niyamas). Upanishads. Vedantic texts conveyed by ancient sages and seers containing their experiences and teachings on the ultimate reality.

Vairagya Non-attachment.

Vaisheshika A treatise on the subtle, causal and atomic principles in relation to the five elements.

Vaishnava One who worships Vishnu in the form of Rama, Krishna, Narayana etc.

Vidya Knowledge.

Vijnana Intuitive ability of mind; higher understanding

Vinyasa Steady flow of connected yoga postures linked with breath work in a continuous movement. For example: sun salutation.

Vayu Wind, prana.

Viveka Reasoning and discerning mind; right knowledge or understanding.

Vritti Circular movement of consciousness; mental and modifications described in raja yoga

Yamas In the Yoga Sutras, Patanjali defined five yamas or ways to relate to others — moral conduct. They are nonviolence; truth and honesty; nonstealing; moderation; and nonpossessiveness.

Yantra Visual form of mantra used for concentration and meditation

Yoga Derived from the Sanskrit word for "yoke" or "join together." Essentially, it means union. It is the science of uniting the individual soul with the cosmic spirit.

Yoga nidra Technique of yogic or psychic sleep which induces deep relaxation

Yogi Someone who practices yoga.

Yogini A female yoga practitioner.

Lightning Source UK Ltd.
Milton Keynes UK
UKHW012354250522
403550UK00002B/50